RECIPES 4 RAW FOOD

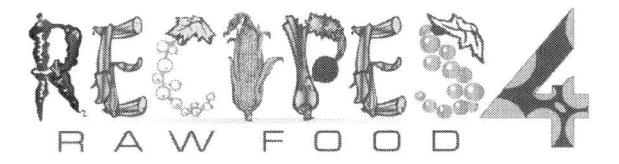

Awesome Raw Food Guide

From how to setup your raw kitchen to the importance of a good yoga practice!

By Kathy Tennefoss

Over 40 New Raw Food Recipes!

Raw Food Recipes & Tips for Living a Healthy Life!

MEMBER OF THE RAW FOODS ASSOCIATION

RECIPES 4
RAW FOOD

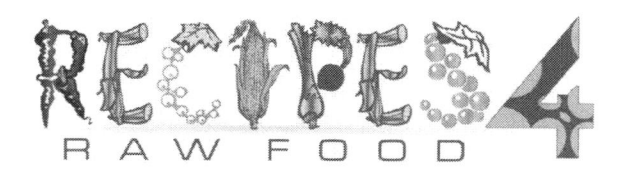

Awesome Raw Food Guide

Sunny Cabana Publishing, L.L.C.

New Orleans, LA70115

www.sunnycabanapublishing.com

By Kathy Tennefoss

All Rights Reserved © 2011 by Kathy Tennefoss

No part of this book may be reproduced or transmitted in any form by any means, graphic, electronic, or mechanical, including photocopying, recording, taping, or by any information storage or retrieval system, without permission in writing from the publisher.

Published by Kathleen Tennefoss
Printed in the United States of America
Author: Kathy Tennefoss
Contributing Author: Mary Rosi
Editor: Shawn M Tennefoss
13-digit ISBN: 9781936874125
10-digit ISBN: 1936874121
First Printing

This book is dedicated to my dad James Kelley for pushing me in the right direction regarding healthy eating, living a healthy active life, and to my loving husband Shawn Tennefoss for suffering through my computer difficulties and taking the time to show me how to orchestrate this book along with sharing his life and journey with me.

Cover design: Kathy & Shawn Tennefoss
Contributing Author Mary Rosi

First edition, 2011

Acknowledgements:

Thanks to everyone who encouraged and inspired me and gave me excellent input and feedback in the raw food industry, including one of my many sisters Heather McNerney, my husband Shawn M. Tennefoss, my dad James Kelley, and Melissa Hernandez and her wonderful family! I would like to also add my special thanks to one of the best yoga teachers Mary Rosi, who has helped me with my personal yoga practice and my health and to one of my favorite raw food enthusiasts Ty Cherry. Without everyone's input I would not have finished this book or started other raw food recipe books. I am extremely grateful to everyone.

If you have any suggestions, comments, or corrections please send me an email to recipes4rawfood@yahoo.com.

Disclaimer:
The responsibility for any adverse detoxification effects resulting from using these recipes described lies not with the author or distributors of this book. This book is not intended for medical advice just as suggestion.
Please enjoy these recipes with your friends and family.

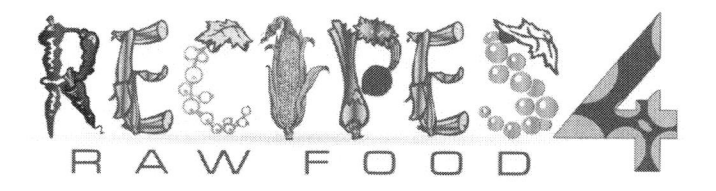

RECIPES 4
RAW FOOD

TABLE OF CONTENTS

Intro Page 7

Some Helpful Tips and Useful Information for Your Raw Kitchen

    Sharp Equipment in the Kitchen Page 15

    What Type Of Juicer Should You Use? Page 21

    What You Should Know About a Dehydrator Page 24

    Raw Food and Sprouting Page 27

    The Right Kind of Oil Page 36

    Raw Coconuts Page 39

    The Sweet and Salty Of Raw Food Page 42

    Turn Up the Heat Page 44

    Raw Nuts Page 46

    The Importance of Yoga for Living a Healthy Life Page 50

Super Smoothies Page 57

Raw Appetizers Page 77

Raw Soups Page 99

Raw Super Salads Page 119

Raw Dinners Page 139

Raw Desserts Page 159

Why Eat Organic Page 181

About The Author Page 184

Other Sources for Raw Food Page 186

Index Page 193

INTRO

I have put together some great raw food recipes that are easy for you and your family to prepare. Making healthy meals together helps to solidify your family values and bring your family closer.

In this raw food book I have gone through only some of my favorite raw recipes that I found are the easiest to make when you are short on time. Everyone is busy but you still should make time to eat a healthy meal. It's also about putting fun into your meals by involving the whole family and have then help and give their input so that they feel like they are contributing to their own health because when your children get older they will remember this and pass the healthy living on to their children. I know this from experience. I had a dad who ate healthy mostly vegetarian meals and biked and a mom who ate only junk food and did not exercise whatsoever. It was a battle at our house of what to eat. I never knew whose food I should eat. It wasn't until I got older and I could choose what and how I should eat.

This is why I feel so compelled to tell others about healthy eating.

I didn't realize until I got older how my dad had influenced me and my food choices. My mom was always sick and did not eat well or take care of herself and that was to her detriment. I vowed to myself and my family that I would try my hardest to seek out the best quality food by purchasing organic produce and by preparing the food as to no lose its nutritional value and I have stuck to that promise for over 20 years. I feel that this has helped me and my family immensely and I want to pass the benefits on to others so that they too will feel that they are contributing to a better healthier way of life.

The raw food diet helps to enable you to lose unwanted pounds, gain muscle tone, facilitate proper digestion, and improve your overall health and appearance. You will be completely revitalized! This approach will help you transform both your body and mind. If you want to achieve real, long lasting results, you must do more than exercise your body. You need to make significant nutritional changes.

Breaking bad eating habits is one of the most challenging things that one can face. You will need to develop good habits that uplift your spirit and bring you happiness through fitness, good health, and mental clarity. Even if your current eating habits are nutritionally sound, here you can find ways to further maximize the benefits of healthy eating.

Learn how to go make raw meals and make healthy decisions. If you choose to email us you'll find we are supportive not judgmental. We can be your guiding light on the road to better health. You will feel better, look better, and have a strong immune system. To experience the joy of nutritional health and vitality the raw food diet will catapult you to the healthy being you want to be!

It has been stated in many natural health and healing books that it is best to drink warm water mixed with 1/2 of a lemon in the morning. I know it's not coffee but it stabilizes the body for the day.

I know that everyone says you need a lot of protein in your diet but you can get your protein from any kind of greens, avocados, olives, coconuts, or flax seeds.

You may notice right away some of the detoxifying effects of eating a raw diet; like loss of energy, diarrhea, headaches, or nausea. When you eat processed and cooked foods it overloads our lymphatic systems, which in turn can cause congestion, illnesses, and colon problems. When you eat a raw food diet it gives your body a rest from digesting cooked food, meat, dairy, or processed foods. Your body needs this time of rest to recoup from all of the bad food choices that we have made in the past like fried foods, sugars, high fat processed foods, etc.

You may also like to take a fiber supplement in the morning and evening which will help clean your colon. I like acia fiber mixed into my smoothies in the morning but you can use whatever you like.

It is also a good idea to exercise along with eating healthy. Even if you just have time for a brisk walk that is better than nothing at all. I prefer yoga because I feel that it helps with many issues within the body along with keeping you fit and that is why I have a small excerpt from one of the best yoga teachers I know but I do enjoy biking and swimming as well. Just find something that you enjoy and stick with it. You will feel better and think more positively about the day.

Please try all of my recipes and put your best foot forward in the fight for obesity, diabetes, heart disease, cancer, and a slew of other ailments that are from not eating a healthy diet. Also remember that life should be fun and that eating healthy doesn't mean that you have to be strict every single day. It's the small efforts that you put forth everyday that make a difference in the long run. People will start to notice your healthy glow and how young you look and start to ask you how, what, and will you show me. This is when you will feel like you have made a difference in the world. So don't waste any more time! Start on your journey to a healthier you!

TIPS AND USEFUL INFORMATION FOR YOUR RAW KITCHEN

SHARP EQUIPMENT IN THE KITCHEN

WHAT TYPE OF JUICER SHOULD YOU USE?

WHAT YOU SHOULD KNOW ABOUT A DEHYDRATOR

RAW FOOD AND SPROUTING

THE RIGHT KIND OF OIL

RAW COCONUTS

THE SWEET AND SALTY OF RAW FOOD

TURN UP THE HEAT

RAW NUTS

THE IMPORTANCE OF YOGA FOR YOUR RAW DIET

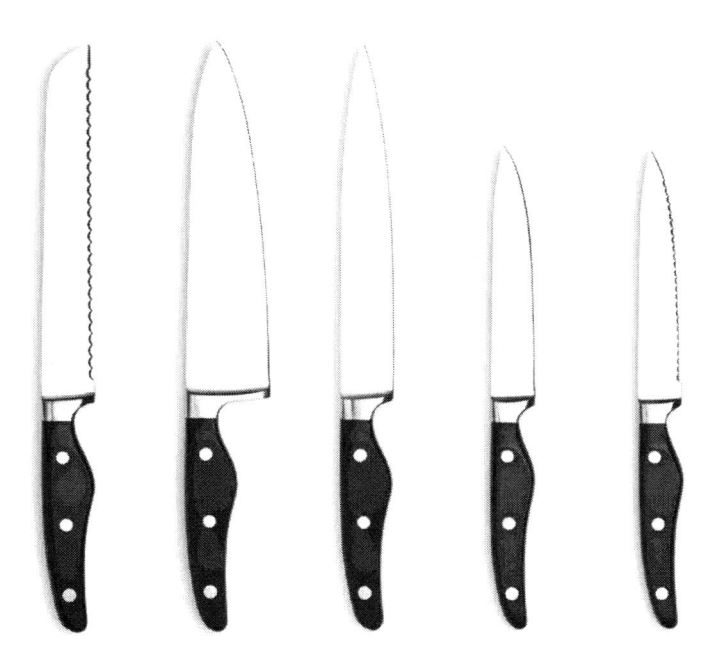

How Important Are Your Cutting Tools In A Raw Kitchen?

Knives are one of the most important parts about a kitchen alongside the produce you are using. You shouldn't overlook their importance because a dull knife can make your experience in the kitchen unbearable. A good set of knives will last much longer and make your life easier in the kitchen plus you won't need to have a cluttered area to work in because you will have your favorite tools right by your side.

There are basically two type of manufacturing of knives: forged and stamped. A forged blade is a piece of hot steel that is pressed into a mold and then hammered into shape. Then the blade is placed between a bolster (wood, etc.). A forged knife usually is thicker and has more flexibility than a stamped knife. Forged blades are usually better quality and are usually more expensive because of their quality. A stamped blade is made out a flat sheet of metal that is sharpened, polished, and shaped into a blade. Stamped blades are thinner and flatter than forged blades.

There are many types of materials that the blades are made with such as, high carbon stainless steel, stainless steel, titanium, ceramic, and plastic. One of my favorites is high carbon stainless steel because they don't tend to rust as much and are a good quality in a blade. Ceramic blades tend to chip or break more easily. The titanium blades are light weight knives that are good for filleting items. The stainless steel blades are also very good but they tend to discolor more often and are harder to keep a sharp edge on them.

One of my favorite knives is a chef's knife. If you can only afford one great knife it would be a chef knife. They usually come in 6 in, 8 in, 10 in, and 12 in sizes. The smaller ones are usually called mini chef knives. One knife that is similar to the chef knife is the santoku knife which is great for cutting vegetables because of the blade is thinner and shorter than a chef knife with scalloped sides. This is another one of my favorites but really the main thing is that the knife has to work well for you. Everyone seems to have their favorite when it comes to knives.

A serrated knife is also a good choice to have on hand. The scalloped sides of the knife make cutting into tomatoes, bread, or anything that is a little softer that you don't want to bruise while slicing and dicing.

Another good knife to have is a paring knife. These usually are small with a curved tip, like a bird on the end of the knife. They are great for cutting, slicing, and putting details on vegetables and fruits, which is sometimes necessary when you have a raw kitchen.

With a raw kitchen there are lots of extra knives and gadgets you could have that may be beneficial like a grapefruit knife, lettuce knife (made of plastic so that it doesn't turn the edges of the lettuce brown when slicing it), peeler, saladacco slicer (hand spiral slicer with different blades for raw zucchini or raw pastas), graters/shredders, zesters, and a garlic press. All of these tools make life a lot easier in the kitchen and make your final product look a little more professional.

Another tool you will need is a wheel knife sharpener or a whetstone. I always keep one on hand. My favorite is a wheel knife sharpener because of the ease in the kitchen.

To keep your knives longer it is best to clean them by hand instead of in the dishwasher. The harsh detergents in the dishwasher tend to dull the knives. Make sure to dry them and put them away in a wooden block. It is also best to use a wooden cutting board when slicing your vegetables and fruits because it creates less resistance than ceramic or plastic cutting boards. Make sure that you clean your board every time you use it because there may be some bacteria left from the garden and it will transfer to your next raw meal.

Over all it's best to make sure that the knives work for you and that they feel good in your hand and are sharp. You don't want to have dull knives because then you have a tendency to slip and cut something more than your fruits and vegetables.

Another one of my favorite sharp items that I keep in my raw kitchen is a Vita Mixer! I could not have a raw kitchen without it. There are so many uses of a Vita Mixer. You can make soups, sauces, dressings, smoothies, etc. I love my Vita Mixer! I could not wake up in the morning without it. I put all kinds of vegetables in the Vita Mixer. Some of these vegetables would be too tough for a regular blender. I know that it is an added expense for a raw kitchen but it is well worth every penny. I even take mine when I travel so that I can eat a healthy meal anywhere! You could just eat a salad to have a raw meal but when you grind up all of your vegetables in a Vita Mixer you end up eating more vegetables and fruits in a single meal. So you are increasing your vitamins, fiber, digestion, nutrients, and health in one meal! It's a great addition to any kitchen even if you are not fully raw! Some things can be made with a blender but if you really want to grind things up smooth get a Vita Mixer.

Another tool of the trade is a food processor. If you have a food processor you can make all kinds of different shapes and sizes of fruits and vegetables for your meals. When you are making raw food you want the appearance to be eye pleasing and with a food processor you can make your meal look more precise. Plus it's' quicker and less work. I sometimes shred my vegetables at the beginning of the week and store them in the refrigerator especially if I know I won't have much time during the week so that I can just grab them and make a raw wrap or salad.

For those who want to add a little more design work to their meals or want to be able to have really think slices it is best to use a mandoline. By using a mandoline you can dice, julienne, thin to thick slices, crinkle cut, waffle cut, diamond, by using different styles of blades. With this you don't need electricity and you can make small or large amounts for your raw kitchen. They can be a little pricy but they are worth every penny if you want a more precise looking cut for your fruits and veggies.

The last thing that I would recommend is a spiral slicer. Spiral slicers are great for making the raw pastas and for nicely decorated salads. It will make anyone look like a professional. You can purchase them online or at most markets.

Choices, Choices, What Type Of Juicer to Use on a Raw Food Diet

These days there is a kitchen appliance to do just about everything. There are choppers, slicers, dicers, juicers, blenders, and much more. With the availability of all these gadgets and gizmos, raw food preparation can be a breeze, not to mention a lot of fun. Let's explore one of these handy tools of the trade:

The raw food juice extractor

A juice extractor provides an excellent way to extract the beneficial nutrients from raw fruits and vegetables. A juicer separates the juice from the pulp of the fruit. Anyone on a raw food diet needs to have a juicer as part of their array of equipment.

There are many different juicers on the market in different price ranges. An electric juicer is much simpler and faster to use than a manual one. There are two main types of juicers:

* Centrifugal (least expensive and the oldest design type) - this type of juicer works using a spinning motion at high speeds. The food is inserted into a chute, and the centrifugal motion spins the juice away from the food fiber. The juice is then dispensed into a separate

container or leaving the pulp fiber behind in a basket. With this type of juicer you can only produce 1-2 quarts before you have to take it apart to clean out the pulp. They also don't juice leafy greens very well, but I have added parsley and cilantro to many of my morning green juices!

* masticating (more expensive but they extract more of the nutrients from the produce) - this juicer works similar to your teeth by grinding and chewing the food fiber while squeezing the juice from the food pulp. This juicer operates at a low speed and has no centrifugal action, and many think it does a more efficient juicing job. You may also use a masticating juicer with a blank plate insert for raw nut butters or raw tomato sauces. You can also grate your vegetables and fruits by not putting a screen or blank in at all.

There are also manual juicers that are used for citrus fruits and leafy greens, such as orange juice or wheat grass.

Centrifugal juice extractors tend to be a lot noisier than masticating juicers. A masticating extractor also tends to make more juice out of less raw food than the spinning type of extractor.

Consider the health benefits of using a juice extractor:

* It's a healthy way to obtain a boost of energy

* Fresh juice is easily absorbed by your body's digestive system

* Fiber is essential for proper nutrition, and raw food juice is an excellent source of it

* Fresh juice without additives or preservatives provides your body with essential minerals, vitamins, and nutrients

* extracting your own juice is much more economical than purchasing at a juice bar

Gazpacho juice drink recipe

Ingredients:

* 2-3 cups of diced ripe tomatoes

* 1 peeled cucumber

* 1 celery stalk, washed and trimmed

* 1-2 green onions, washed and trimmed

* Black pepper, fine grain sea salt, cayenne pepper to taste

* Organic hot sauce (optional)

Directions:

1. Wash and prepare raw food for extraction.

2. Juice the tomatoes, cucumber, celery, green onions, and seasonings.

3. Pour into glass and season with Tabasco if desired.

4. Enjoy!

Dehydrators – A Great Way to Preserve Food!

Since eons, people have preserved food by drying it in the sunlight or shade. This way you can enjoy your favorite foods even when they are not available or it's out of season. Most fruits and vegetables can be dehydrated and preserved for a very long time. Dehydrating food also keeps most of the nutrients in tacked, as if it were just picked!

Most modern homes use an electric dehydrator to dehydrate fruits and vegetables like apples, bananas, grapes, kale, etc. Electric dehydrators do an excellent job at maintaining a better control over the temperature along with dehydrating larger quantities of food at once.

There are different types of electric dehydrators available in the market today. The most useful is the stacker type, where you can stack multiple trays of food according to your need. You can choose from counter top dehydrators or free standing ones depending on the amount of food you need to dehydrate and also the amount of space you have. Some models have a rigid box with removable trays whereas others offer stackable trays. Some models use a fan at the bottom to circulate the hot air whereas others use the convection method. Choose a model, which you like and which is perfect for your dehydrating needs.

You can also make fruit leathers and roll ups by pureeing the fruit and dehydrating it to a leathery state. Another good and fun food choice is to make raw crackers out of seeds and nuts. When dehydrating fruits or vegetables you can add other herbs, spices, seasonings and even honey to make them tastier and more flavorful.

The time taken to dehydrate would depend on the moisture content of the food and the thickness of the slices. The temperatures should be appropriate. If it is too low, you run a risk of spoiling the food on the other hand a high temperature will result in hardening of the surface of the food thus trapping moisture inside. The temperatures should be high enough to draw the moisture from the food and at the same time low enough that the food does not get cooked.

A dehydrator is a great way to preserve food and add more fruit and vegetables to your daily diet. Also you can enjoy your favorite fruits even when they are not available fresh in the market. So eat your fruits and veggies!

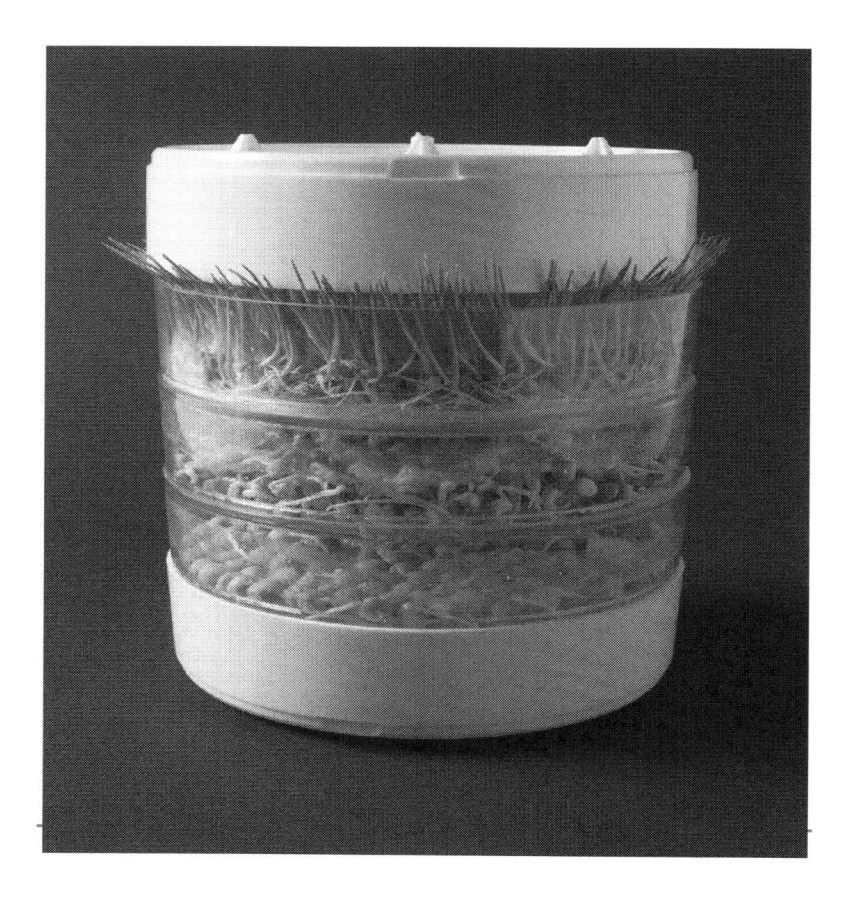

Why Are Sprouts So Healthy For You?

Sprouts have always been a favorite among those who have looked for a healthy diet. But exactly why are sprouts so good for you? Why are they healthier than the seeds themselves?

The simple reason is that the seed is now preparing for a new life. The germination process changes the in nutritive value of the seeds.

The ascorbic acid and vitamin c content of the seed increases substantially with only forty-eight hours of germination. B complex, and the vitamins riboflavin, biotin and niacin also increase by the germination process. The only disadvantage is that the folic acid content comes down.

Sprouts are a great source of concentrated minerals, vitamins and enzymes. They are inexpensive and easily made at home. When the seed sprouts most of the starch is converted into simple sugars. Thus sprouts are basically a predigested food form. Sprouts are also extremely high in fiber content.

The sprouting process can be easily done at home. All you need to do is soak the seeds for a few hours. The time would depend on the type of seed you would like to sprout. Soft seeds like alfalfa need to be soaked for short-time where as hard seeds like fenugreek and lentils need to be soaked for over 12 hours. Do make sure that all of the seeds and nuts that you sprout are raw! Nuts and seeds that have been roasted are unable to sprout due to the fact that they have been heated to a high temperature.

Once the seeds are soft from soaking, there are a few methods that you can use to sprout them. You can tie them into a muslin cloth, place in a vessel and keep in a dark place. You can also put them into a jar and cover the mouth with a muslin cloth and leave them to sprout. Remember to use a jar, which can hold 4-5 times the volume of seeds. You can also use a plastic sprouter, which has two to three separators so that you may sprout different seeds at the same time. Make sure you drain and rinse the water every 6-8 hours. Once you have done that and they have sprouted expose them to light for around 6 hours to activate the chlorophyll.

Sprouting your own healthy seeds in a healthy raw food diet is not only convenient, but also saves money on your grocery bill. Seed sprouting is not difficult, even if you don't consider yourself to have a green thumb. Sprouting your own seeds is easy, healthy, and economical.

Here are a few points to ponder regarding a sprout starter for your kitchen:

* You can sprout many different varieties of seeds, so there's always variety in your raw food diet.

* You can choose a sprout starter that suits your specific needs. There are small single tier models, multi-tiered stackable sprouting systems, or you can use a glass mason jar.

* You can choose totally organic seeds for your sprout starter.

* Sprouts are very healthy and loaded with beneficial nutrients, digestive enzymes, minerals, protein, amino acids, vitamins, and iron.

* It only takes a few days to have sprouts from your starter.

* the growing season for sprouts is year round, and you can grow them no matter what the climate is where you live.

* just a few of the sprouts you can grow in a starter include mung beans, green peas, clover, lentils, alfalfa, almonds, sunflower, radish, buckwheat, wheat, cabbage, kale, quinoa, sesame, broccoli, snow peas, and garbanzo beans.

* fresh organic sprouts go straight from sprouter to table, so you enjoy nutritious sprouts that have not been sitting for an unknown length of time on a grocery shelf. Your sprouts are always fresh, coming straight out of your starter to be rinsed and instantly enjoyed.

Different types of sprout starters

There are commercial sprout starters available or you can simply create your own. Commonly used methods for sprouting include:

* Glass mason jars

* Cloth

* Plastic tubes

* Plastic mesh

* Clay saucers

* Plastic trays

* Hemp bags

Fresh sprouts are one of the healthiest and most nutritious foods you can include in your organic raw food diet. By growing your own sprouts, you are assured of having fresh organic sprouts handy whenever you want them. You can omit chemicals, pesticides, and synthetic fertilizers so the sprouts you grow are 100% organic.

Sprout salad extravaganza

Ingredients:

* Fresh spinach leaves

* Diced cucumbers

* halved cherry tomatoes

* Sunflower greens

* Buckwheat lettuce

* Sprouts grown from a bean blend

* Sea salt and fresh ground black pepper

* Oil and vinegar

Directions:

1. Clean and prepare greens, vegetables, and sprout ingredients.

2. Toss together with salt, pepper, and oil and vinegar dressing.

3. Enjoy!

HERE IS A LIST OF FEW SEEDS THAT YOU SPROUT AT HOME AND USE IN DIFFERENT RECIPES.

SPROUT	SOAKING TIME IN HRS	SPROUTING TIME IN DAYS
ALFALFA	5-10	3-5
AMARNATH	5-10	3-5
SOY BEANS	8-10	2-3
ADZUKI BEANS	9-12	2-3
CHICKPEAS	9-12	2-3

MUNG BEANS	9-12	2-3
SOYBEANS	9-12	2-3
BROCCOLI	9-12	2-3
BUCKWHEAT	10-12	2-3
FLAX SEEDS	4-6	3-4
CORN	10-15	3-5
SESAME	4-6	2-4
GREEN LENTILS	10-12	2-3
RED LENTILS	10-12	2-3

MILLET	8-11	1-2
QUINOA	8-10	2-3
RADISH	8-10	2-3
RYE	9-12	2-4
SUNFLOWER	6-8	2-3
RED WHEAT	10-12	7-10
WHEAT BERRIES	10-12	7-10
BARLEY	8-14	2-3

OATS	8-14	2-3
RICE	12-18	1-2
ALMOND	10-14	1-2
CABBAGE	6-14	1-2
FENUGREEK	8-14	18 HRS
PUMPKIN	8-14	1-2
PEANUT	12-14	1-2

Sprouts are best eaten raw. You can make salads or sandwich spreads using sprouts. They taste really good when you add chopped tomatoes, onions and bell peppers along with salt and lemon juice. Sprouts can also be steamed or cooked for consumption but they retain their nutritive value best in raw state.

The Right Kind of Oil

There are so many different types of oils out there. Which ones are the best for your health and which ones taste the best? It is always best to buy fresh organic oils if you can. They taste better and are better for you. Oils that are pressed from fruits, nuts, and seeds are to most nutritional.

When you are purchasing oils try to buy the best quality that you can afford. It is also a good idea to purchase in small quantities and double check the use by date. If you have a larger budget it is also fun to purchase different types of oils for a change of flavor. It is also best to store your oils in a tightly closed, cool, and dark place to reduce the rate of oxidation. If it smells fishy it probably needs to be thrown out. Some even say that oils such as avocado, walnut, and peanut should be stored in the refrigerator to lessen their oxidation.

It seems like when you are at the supermarket and you are in the oil and vinegar aisle that there are endless choices. It takes almost as long to pick out the oil as it does to drive to the store. Should you buy first pressing, cold pressed, and what is extra virgin? Well the oils with the most flavors are the first pressing without heat. So sometimes you will see on the label first pressing cold pressed this is usually the best quality and flavor. Extra virgin is the first cold pressed oil that has less contaminant because it is from the middle of the cold pressing where the oil is flowing heavily. Extra virgin oil is the best quality and flavor. There is still more oil left within the fruit for 2-3 more pressing using heat. This produces lighter less healthy oil.

Using heat to extract oils can be harmful to the body and usually has free radicals, which can cause cellular damage. A good organic olive oil can improve your skin, nails, hair, digestion, and your overall energy.

I always try to choose organic extra virgin olive oil for my salads and for my raw food recipes. If you eat your salad without good oil it's like getting dressed up for a night out without jewelry or makeup. So experiment with cold pressed, organic oils for your next salad or recipe! Your family will love the flavor and the health benefits.

One of my favorite oils that I use every day is hemp oil. I use this in my smoothies because there are so many health benefits and hemp oil has a great nutty flavor!

Hemp seeds or oil is considered a "perfect food" for humans due to its ideal 3:1 linoleic acid (la-omega 6) to alpha linolenic acid (lna-omega 3) ratio hemp oil provides the body with an ideal balance of essential fatty acids (efa's). With the ability to provide every vital efa for the entirety of a human life there is no other raw food or oil that can match hemp's efficiency and value in regards to this aspect of health. Low in saturated fatty acids hemp is the only oil that does not cause acid deficiencies through continual and focused use within an appropriate diet. Also conducive to frozen storage over long periods of time, unlike other oils it is not susceptible to rapid nutrient deterioration and does not require preservatives for increased shelf life. If manufactured and processed right everything about hemp is natural and from the earth which is received well by our bodies. Some of the health benefits of hemp oil include but are not limited to more vibrant skin, increased endurance, inflammation reduction, water retention, better blood pressure, immune system improvement, pain reduction, weight loss and much more. It can also help with diseases like arthritis, cancer and those relating to the heart. In addition to the essential fatty acids mentioned above hemp oil delivers essential amino acids, the rare protein globule edestins and gamma-linolenic acid (gla-omega 6) and stearidonic acid (sda-omega 3) all of which are crucial to the proper functioning of the body. Hemp is a truly wondrous raw food that should never be ignored. If you are currently not aware of all the benefits of hemp and hemp seed oil it is certainly a subject that you would be wise to research more thoroughly. Raw food enthusiasts often overlook its value due to some of the miss-informed stigmas attached to the product.

Hemp seeds are 35% protein, 47% fat, and 12% carbohydrates. Hempseeds are packed full of protein, which is helpful to build your body's muscles, tendons, organs, hair, nails, etc. This is especially good for raw, vegan, and vegetarian diets. Hempseeds contain all the essential amino acids and essential fatty acids that are necessary to sustain life. It is increasingly used as a dietary option by those who understand raw food and even by those who are simply looking for a way to live healthier.

RAW COCONUTS

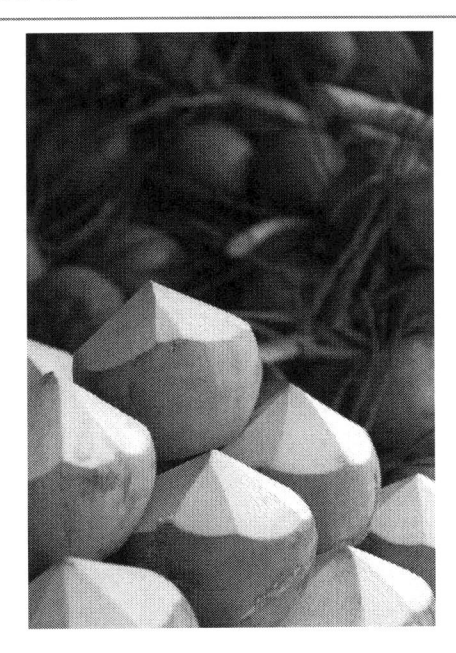

IF YOU ARE NOT SURE ABOUT HOW TO USE A RAW YOUNG COCONUT HERE IS AN EASY SOLUTION FOR YOU.

Young coconuts are not just a wonderful delicacy. There are so many ways in which young coconuts do wonders for our health like lowering cholesterol, reduce the risk of heart disease, and has anti-inflammatory benefits for the body.

In the tropical region it is considered to be the most important fruit, simply because people know of its medicinal properties and also because of its mineral rich water, such as potassium, copper, iron, calcium, ascorbic acid, and b-complex vitamins. Young coconuts are highly nutritious in nature and have medicative qualities, which are very good for your heart, liver and kidneys. In fact, the latest research reports suggest that apart from its nutritional features the young coconuts are reported to reduce the viral load of human immuno-deficiency virus or HIV.

It's also known for its natural electrolyte source. Also, it is believed that many people living in third world countries have actually been saved by these young coconuts. The coconuts in their young age happen to be the most health enhancing. Not to mention the fact that it's similar to blood plasma and has been used in emergency blood transfusions.

These are just few of the benefits of young coconuts. Now let's discuss how to open and eat a young coconut as many people find this a tough job to do:

The best and simplest way to open a coconut is to put the coconut inside a plastic bag, tie its ends and just swing it on any flat, hard surface, which would shatter the young coconut into shards. You can get the meat simply by separating coconut meat from the husk in this fashion. Use the plastic bag to retain the coconut water. Now hold the plastic bag so that the liquid settles down at the bottom. You can now puncture a hole and get a glassful of coconut juice. It's as easy as 1, 2, 3. .

The meats of young coconut are quite soft and can be scooped out with a spoon or a knife. However, the suggested way is to use a small knife with a flexible blade, which would allow it to follow the contour of the shell while undercutting the meat out of the shell.

The young coconuts are great choice for the summers as they quite easy to prepare and they are available at most grocery store. Young coconuts are a great enhancer to various drinks, especially tropical drinks, smoothies, pies, and dinner dishes as well. Humid countries rely heavily on coconut-based foods.

The Sweet and Salty of Raw Food

For the most part you will eventually use some type of natural sweeteners or salty flavoring for your raw food recipes. Using refined sugars are not beneficial to the body because sugar imbalances the body gives you an energy crash. Companies have been trying to manufacture sweeteners like saccharine and aspartame, which have reports of being taken off the market for being toxic or causing cancer, either way it doesn't sound that great when there are tons of natural alternatives out there in the supermarket.

Most food in its raw state is flavorful without it but when you are trying to make a recipe with combined ingredients you will want to use either celtic salt, himalayan salt (this is one of my favorites due to the great mineral content), or other flavored salts that they have on the market. You can also use a product called Braggs liquid amino acids (which you can purchase in most health food stores) as a salt substitute. Braggs has many amino acids and enzymes that are necessary for your body to function properly and it is not fermented. You may also use a product that is called nama shoyu, which is a raw fermented soy sauce for flavoring many dishes.

As far as sweet goes one of my favorite sweeteners to use is agave (cactus) nectar. I use it in smoothies and in my green tea but there are many other ways to sweeten your raw food. You can use date sugar (or if you don't have date sugar you may use just plain dates) which, is made of ground up dried dates and by using date sugar you have added fiber to your recipe. What a bonus! You can also use other dried fruits that are ground up in a food processor. You will just have to experiment to see what you like best. Raw honey is also another great choice. I have used this on occasion. Raw honey is honey that has not been heated during the extraction from the hive. By using raw honey you will also have the benefits of enzymes, b-complex, and minerals. Another one of my favorites is maple syrup because it mixes well in liquids and has tons of minerals and a great flavor. Turbinado sugar is another good choice that is made from partially refined raw sugar which can be better if you want a smoother finish in a dessert or smoothie.

So all in all you won't really miss refined sugar or table salt if you just follow the above choices for your now and future recipes. Plus you are adding more minerals, fiber, enzymes, and amino acids to your diet. So life can be sweeter and for you folks that like things a little salty try some new ways of flavoring your meals.

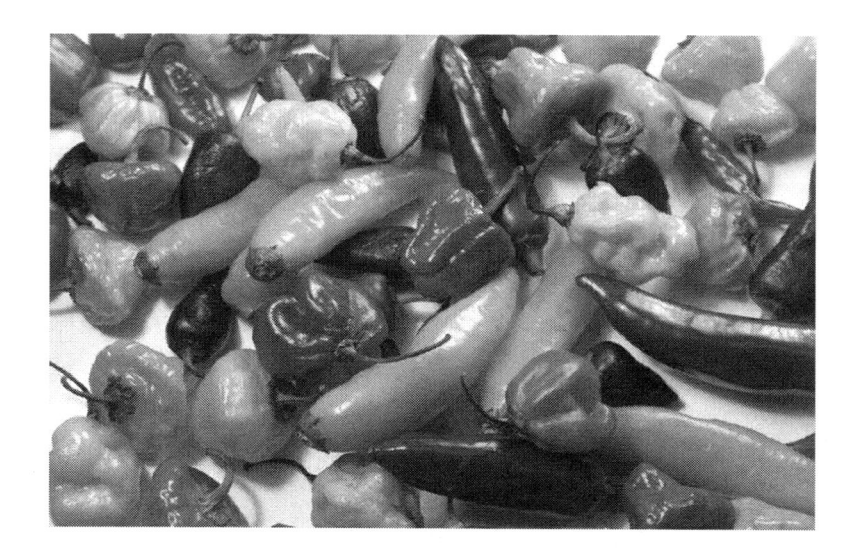

Turn Up the Heat

There are many ways to make your raw food dishes spicy. Here are some of my favorites: jalapenos, habanera, serrano, banana, scotch bonnet, Thai peppers, chilies, cayenne, and the list goes on. There are over 20 varietals of peppers and not all of them are hot but they do add tons of flavor to dishes. You can use these in their raw state or dehydrated state for your recipes. Either way they will both taste great and add tons of flavor, color, and health benefits. Just remember that a little goes a long way! It is also a good idea to use gloves when cutting them so that you won't forget later and rub your eyes because some of those peppers can be very potent.

Peppers are beneficial to the body because they have vitamin a, c, and k plus a good amount of fiber. Peppers help prevent cell damage, inflammation, asthma, cancer, decrease cholesterol, reduce ulcers, support immune function and can help with weight loss. They only have between 10-20 calories per serving but they add so much flavor and so many health benefits to your body. How can you not love them?

Other ways to make dishes spicy is by adding raw garlic, ginger, basil, horseradish, onions, or seaweed. All of these are so beneficial for your body as well. Garlic has been known to be a powerful natural antibiotic and there have been studies that have shown that garlic has reduced ones cholesterol. Ginger is another great addition to anyone's diet. Ginger helps with upset stomachs, nausea, and poor digestion. A couple of benefits of eating basil are that it has been known to help with nausea and motion sickness. Horseradish has c and b-complex vitamins and has been used to treat such illnesses as toothache, scurvy, coughs, aching joints, and diabetes. Onions have been used to treat colds, coughs, and asthma. Seaweed or sea vegetables have so many benefits for the body and there are so many different varietals that I can't even begin talk about them. Dulse is one of my favorites and makes a great addition to salads and raw soups.

You will find many health benefits and have a blast trying new recipes with all of these different ways to spice up your meals. There are so many benefits to making your dishes spicy why wouldn't you spice it up a bit? Spice it up for you and your family's health.

Raw Nuts

I also wanted to include some information on the benefits of nuts since they are in a lot of my recipes and are considered a staple in the raw food diet.

Almost all of the desserts have nuts in them and I think that it would be good for you to know some of the benefits of the nuts for you and your family.

Nuts are an amazing food. Nuts are very beneficial for your health and they taste great too! Nuts are high in calories but they are still very beneficial to your body because they are loaded with mono saturated fats, which help to lower heart disease. Many nuts are rich in omega 3 fatty acids. Omega 3 essential fatty acids are good for your heart and for your arteries. Omega 3 essential fatty acids are helpful for making your heart rhymes more stable so you can try to avoid a heart attack. Nuts also have l-arginine which is helpful to your heart and arteries because it makes your arteries more flexible and leads to less blood clots. Nuts also have been known to have plant sterols in them which help to lower cholesterol.

It is best to eat nuts raw, soaked, or sprouted because they are considered to be live foods. Live foods are foods that have not been heated at high temperatures or cooked. Heating nuts to above 118 degrees starts to destroy beneficial enzymes. When these enzymes are destroyed the nuts are unable to sprout so they would be considered not live.

Some of the best raw nuts are walnuts, cashews, Brazil, macadamia, almonds, pecans, and filberts. They also make great milks when processed correctly. Almonds are one of my favorite nuts they are high in protein, vitamin e, magnesium, zinc, potassium, and iron. Almonds also have the highest amount of calcium of any other nut so they make a great substitute for dairy products for raw foodist and vegans. Almonds also have some of the highest fiber content of any other nut. Cashews are another good nut but should be refrigerated once the package is opened because the spoil easily. Cashews are high in copper and magnesium. Cashews also have one of the lowest fat content of any other nut. Macadamia nuts are also one of my favorites. Macadamia nuts are a high energy food and contain no cholesterol. The natural oils in macadamias contain 78% monounsaturated fats, the highest of any oil including olive oil. Macadamias contain tocopherols and tocotrienols, which are derivatives of vitamin e, phytosterols such as sitosterol and also selenium. One of the best nuts for your health are walnuts. Walnuts are one of the best sources of omega 3 essential fatty acids and they have more antioxidants than most other nuts. Brazil nuts are extremely nutrient rich and high in antioxidants like selenium which helps to neutralize free radicals. Filberts are also very beneficial. If you add filberts to your salads or smoothies then they help you to absorb the fat soluble vitamins a, d, e, and k. Filberts are also great for anti aging properties such as Alzheimer's, stroke, arthritis, wrinkles, and heart disease.

Almost all nuts have photo nutrients which are biologically active components that protect our bodies systems. Many nuts act as antioxidants, which scavenge the free radicals that oxidize blood fats. Photo nutrients operate as part of complex systems that are only partly understood.

Nuts are an amazing food! They are so good for you and they taste great and can be used in so many raw and vegan recipes but just be careful to not over eat them because they are high in calories.

The Importance of Yoga with Your Raw Diet

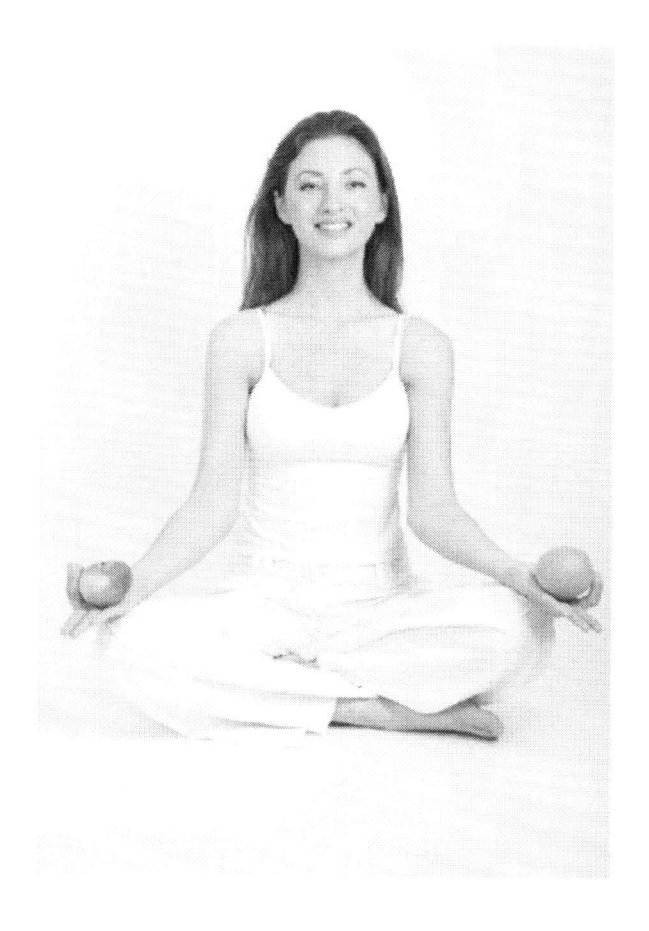

Asana – Yoga on the Mat - Proper Exercise

"One should practice asanas that make one firm, free of diseases, and light of limb."

~Hatha Yoga Pradipika~

There are many types of exercise, but the Yoga system of asana "steady poses" with breath is complete. It emphasizes mental focus, breathing and flowing movements. It is designed to promote mental focus and physical well-being. The steady postures free the mind from disturbances promoting a steadiness and balance that can be brought into one's life beyond the mat. With continuous practice of movement with breath, your asana work will have the same effect as acupuncture or shiatsu, but over time will last longer. The different postures open up lines of energy in the body that respond to the physical, emotional and spiritual aspect of the yogi. The aim of all Yoga practice is to achieve truth wherein the individual soul identifies itself with a higher consciousness. As the mind develops, the veil covering the soul becomes thinner and the soul realizes its identification with a Higher Being. This is the aim of all Yoga. Yoga is a scientific way to bring about this evolution where there is no duality, no subject or object, where the knower, the knowledge, and the known are fused into one. Through this knowledge....peace, strength and well-being are brought about.

~*Neem Karoli Baba*~Yoga is a way of life that integrates the education of your body, your mind & your spirit. To the ancient Yogis, the body was seen as a vehicle for the soul. Just as a car requires that all systems run efficiently, so the body has needs for it to function smoothly.

Food has two purposes for the Yogi...fuel for energy and raw material to repair itself. When digested, this fuel will break down into usable forms and be transported to all the cells of our bodies. Fiber, protein, fats, carbohydrates, vitamins & minerals are essential to the body as a whole for it to function at its best.

In the Yoga Sutras, Patanjali compiled findings of ancient Yogis who studied the many obstacles to bringing the mind under conscious control. He describes eight limbs to the science of Yoga, with the first being the Yamas – truth, non-violence, non-stealing. This limb is expressed in many ways in the Yoga practice. One of the ways is a vegetarian diet. The first of the Yamas is to practice non-injury to all living things and is extended to include non-injury to the planet as well. We need to respect the earth and the animals. The fear and the pain of a slaughtered animal is taken into our bodies when we eat meat. My Guru once told someone when asked why he doesn't eat meat and he said 'I don't eat fear'.

The Yoga scriptures divide food into three types. Sattvic -pure, rajasic-stimulating, & tamasic-impure. Foods that are rajasic are over-stimulating like coffee, tea, tobacco, fast foods, snacks. Foods that are tamasic make one lethargic like meat, drugs, alcohol, packaged foods. Sattvic foods that calm the mind and sharpen the intellect are without preservatives or anything artificial. They are ideally in the form of raw and consist of fresh fruits & vegetables, pure juices, grains, legumes, nuts, seeds, honey, fresh herbs, salads, and raw dairy products.

A sattvic diet brings purity and calmness to the mind and body. It is easily digested and supplies maximum energy. It also helps to minimize fatigue. Yogis believe that people's food preferences reflect their mental clarity and can alter one's spiritual development.

Om Shanti Peace ~ Parvati
www.yogaearth.org

Mary Rosi...(561) 374-3330
Prana Body
7400 N Federal Hwy Ste A5
Boca Raton, FL
www.yoga earth.org
Yoga E-RYT, Teacher Trainer
Reiki Teacher
Certified Iridologist
Aromatherapy
Herbology
Thai Yoga Master

Just as raw food heals the body so does yoga by eliminating toxins and increasing your strength, balance, flexibility, and mind. Yoga also helps with lowering blood pressure, promotes weight loss, strengthens bones, improves immune functions, lowers stress, lowers blood sugar, improves cholesterol, and increase oxygen supply to the tissues.

You should start slowly if you haven't done yoga before or with a good yoga instructor and please check with your doctor before performing any exercise routine because it is better to check first then to find out later. Also be careful when transitioning in and out of poses because that is where most yoga injuries happen. Make sure to take yoga slowly or to your capacity level. You will eventually get straighter, more flexible, and stronger. It could take months or even years but be patient it will pay off in the long run.

Yoga has helped me to stand straighter, be more focused, and much stronger. I could not do a lot of the yoga poses when I first started but now that I am stronger I can do much more. The thing about yoga is that you don't really know you are getting stronger and getting taller it gradually happens and you start to feel better about yourself and life. Yoga helps to reduce stress in your life by focusing your mind on the poses and by releasing toxins that are in your body through breathing and yoga poses.

Incorporating yoga with your raw food diet will make your body run more efficiently which will benefit you in the short and long run. Some have said that yoga helps with alcoholism, anxiety, arthritis, back, cancer, diabetes, heart disease, high blood pressure, insomnia, menopausal disorders, migraines, obesity, and even smoking. So why wouldn't you try it! If you are already eating a healthy diet by adding more raw food than why wouldn't you at least try to add yoga to your routine? You don't have to do yoga everyday but at least try it you may like it! I love yoga and feel that there are so many benefits that I can't possibly list them all. Sometimes just doing downward facing dog for a couple minutes will give you inspiration for your day ahead.

Even if you decide not to participate in yoga it is still a good idea to get some type of exercise into your daily routine. Going for a walk, weight lifting, aerobics, biking, swimming, or running are also good alternatives for getting your daily exercises. Yoga will also help with these daily activities as well by making you more balanced and stronger during these activities.

Super Smoothies

POPEYE'S GREEN MACHINE

STRAWBERRY GREEN MACHINE

GREENELOUPE

WHAT THE KALE

MANGO MAMMA

ACAI SUPER CHARGER

PEACHES & GREEN

GREEN APPLE

GREEN KIWI

CUCUMBER MADNESS

CHOCOLATE HEAVEN

TROPICAL PAPAYA

SWEET CHERRY

GREEN TEA SMOOTHIE

BLUEBERRY GINGER SMOOTHIE

PEAR SMOOTHIE

GREEN NECTARINE

BLACKBERRY DREAM

MIXED GREEN BERRY

FIGLISIOUS

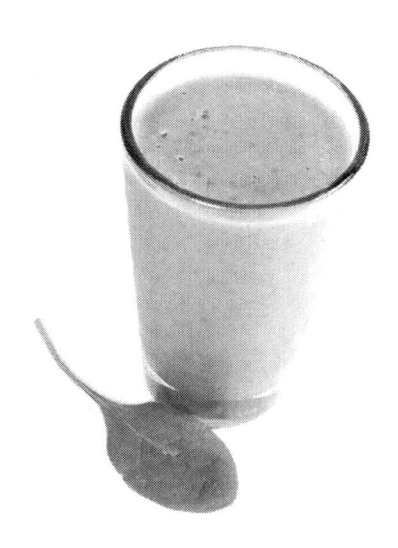

POPEYE'S GREEN MACHINE

1 cup almond milk

2 cups spinach

¼ cup aloe vera juice

1 scoop raw meal replacement (I use garden of life)

1 cup blueberries

Splash of lime juice

1 cup of ice

Mix this all in a vita mixer or blender and serve. This makes two small glasses or one large glass.

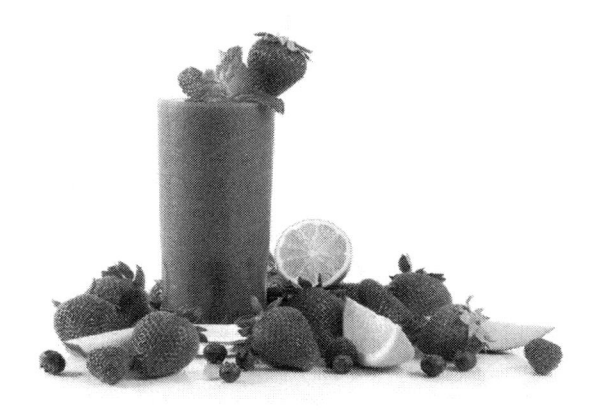

STRAWBERRY GREEN DREAM

1 cup almond milk

1 cup spinach

1 cup celery

¼ aloe vera juice

1 scoop raw meal replacement

1 cup strawberries

¼ cup lime juice

1 cup of ice

Mix all the ingredients in a vita mixer and a blender and serve. This makes two glasses or one large glass.

GREENELOUPE

2 cups celery

1 cup almond milk

1 cup cantaloupe

¼ cup lime juice

1 cup of ice

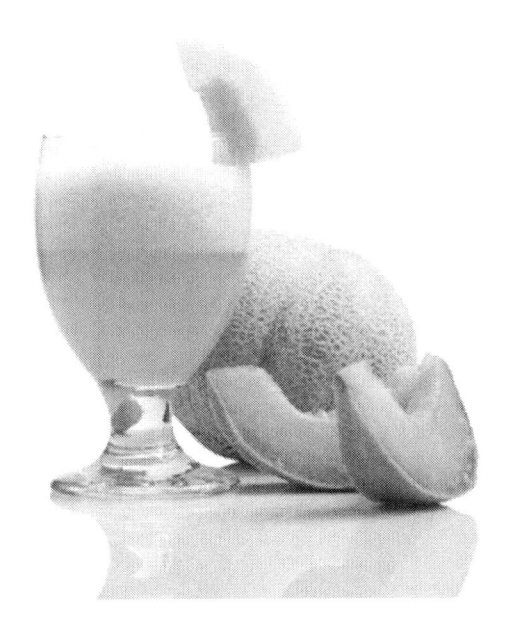

Mix all ingredients in a vita mixer or blender and serve. This makes two medium glasses.

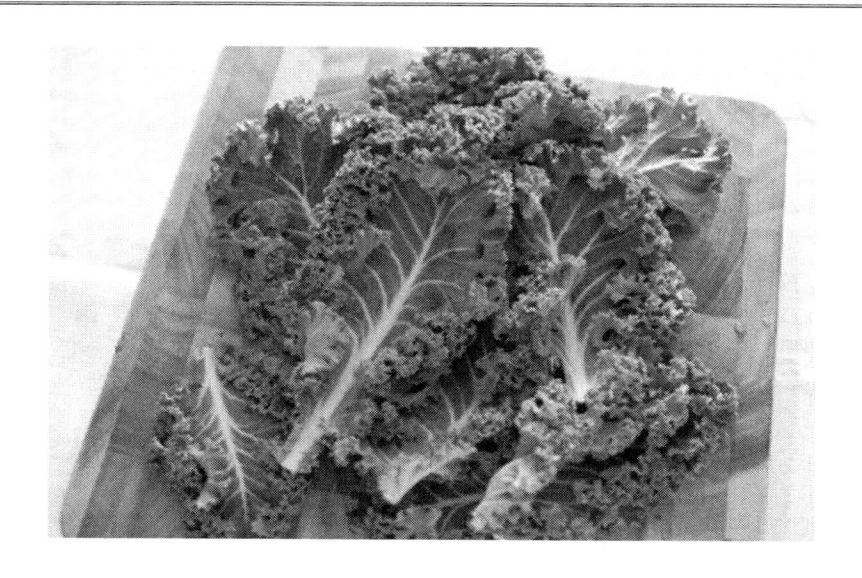

WHAT THE KALE

2 cups green kale

1 frozen banana (when your bananas start to get to ripe its best to peel them and slice them in smaller pieces so that you can use them later in smoothies)

1 cup almond milk

5-7 medium strawberries

1 cup blueberries

1 scoop raw food meal replacement

1 cup of ice

Mix ingredients in a vita mixer or blender and serve. This makes two medium glasses.

MANGO MAMMA

1 cup frozen mangos (you can use fresh if you have it but the consistency will be a little thinner)

2 cups of celery

½ cup almond milk

½ Cup orange juice

½ frozen banana

1 scoop of raw meal replacement

1 seeded date

1 tablespoon coconut oil

1 cup of ice

Blend all ingredients in a vita mixer or blender and serve. This makes two large glasses.

ACIA SUPER CHARGER

1 small package of frozen acia berry (you can purchase this in most super markets or health food stores)

2 cups spinach

1 cup blueberries

½ cup almond milk

1 small orange peeled and cut into quarters

1 scoop of raw meal replacement

1 cup of ice

1 tablespoon of coconut oil

1 pitted date

Mix all ingredients in a vita mixer or blender and serve. This makes 2 medium glasses.

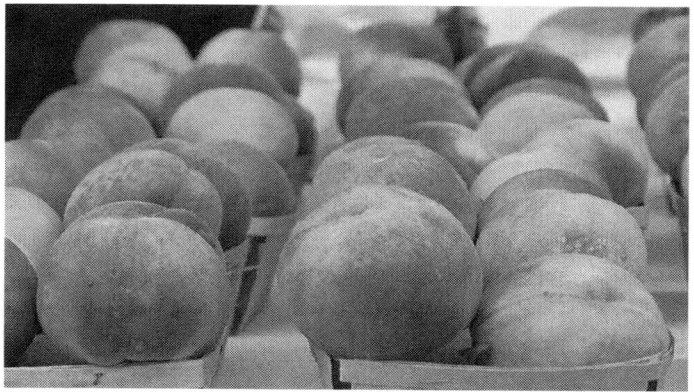

PEACHES & GREEN

2 small peaches with the pit removed and cut into quarters

2 cup romaine lettuce

1 cup celery

¾ cup of orange juice

1 scoop raw meal replacement

1 cup of ice

Mix all ingredients in a vita mixer or a blender and serve. This makes two medium glasses.

GREEN APPLE

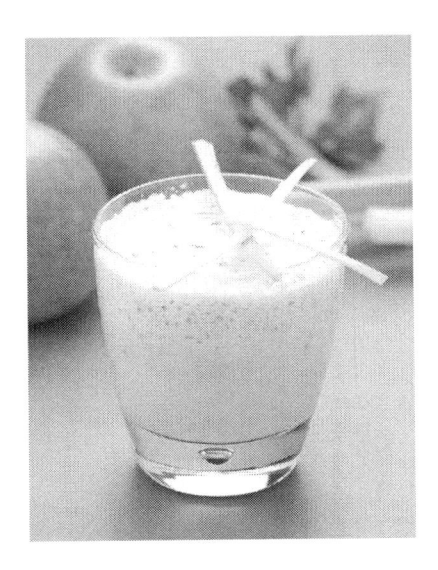

2 cups spinach

1 green apple seeded and cut into quarters

¼ cup lime juice

1 cup almond milk

1 scoop raw meal replacement

1 cup of ice

Mix all ingredients in a vita mixer or blender and serve. This makes two small glasses.

GREEN KIWI

1 cup spinach

1 cup celery

4 kiwis peeled and cut

½ cup lime juice

½ cup almond milk

½ cup orange juice

1/8 cup aloe vera juice

1 scoop raw meal replacement

1 cup of ice

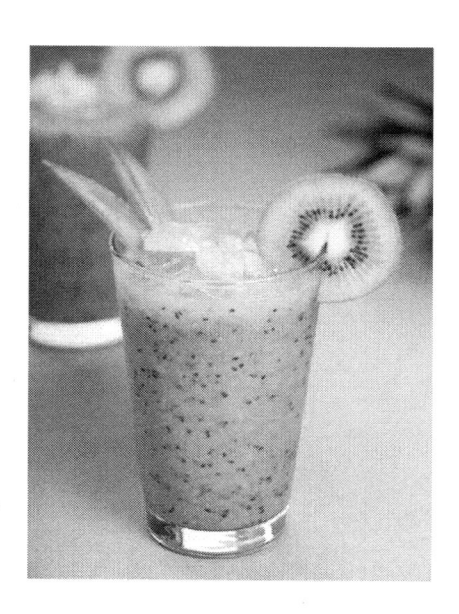

Mix all ingredients in a vita mixer or blender and serve. This makes 2 medium glasses.

CUCUMBER MADNESS

1 large cucumber peeled

1 hass avocado

¼ cup lime juice

1 cup water

1 cup ice

½ bunch of flat leaf parsley

Mix all ingredients together in a vita mixer or blender and serve. This makes two small glasses.

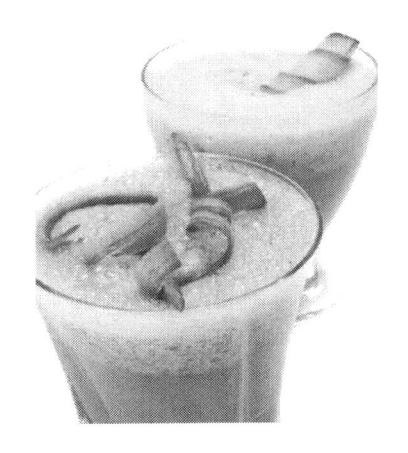

CHOCOLATE HEAVEN

1 hass avocado (pitted and sliced)

3 tablespoons of raw cocoa powder

1 tablespoon of agave nectar

1 tablespoon of coconut

2 dates pitted

2 cups almond milk

1 cup of ice

1 frozen banana

Mix all ingredients in a vita mixer or blender and serve. This is a great treat!

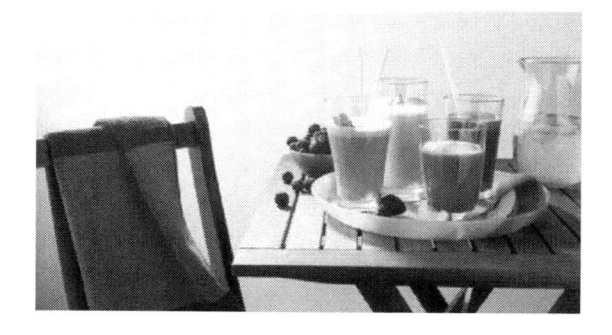

TROPICAL PAPAYA

1 ½ cups papaya

½ cup pineapple

1 frozen banana

1 cup coconut milk

1 cup

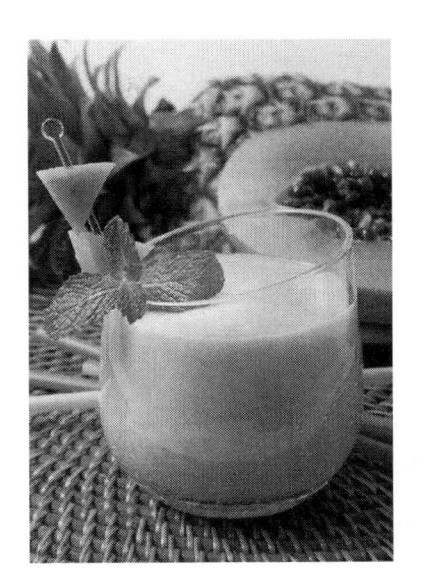

Mix all ingredients in a vita mixer or blender and serve. This is another yummy treat!

SWEET CHERRY

1 cup frozen cherries

2 cups romaine lettuce

1 orange peeled and cut into quarters

1 cup almond milk

1 cup ice

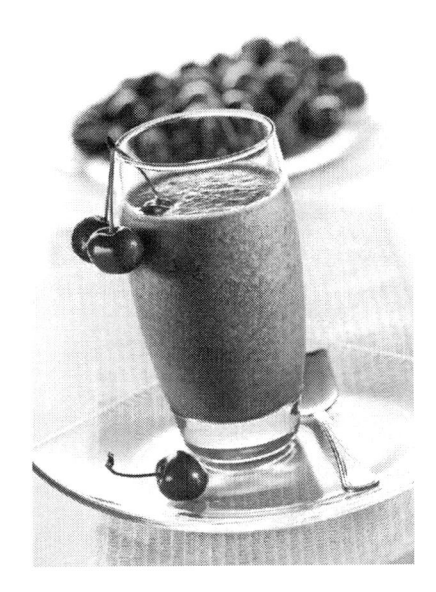

Splash of lime juice

Mix all ingredients in a vita mixer or blender and serve. This makes two small glasses.

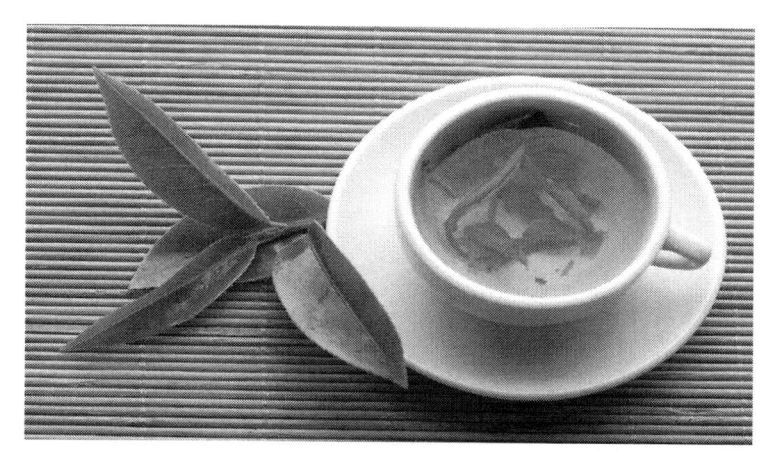

GREEN TEA SMOOTHIE

1 ½ cups of chilled green tea

1 cup almond milk

1 cup of romaine lettuce

1 date pitted

1 cup of ice

Mix all ingredients in a vita mixer or blender and serve. This is a nice and refreshing drink in the summer!

BLUEBERRY GINGER SMOOTHIE

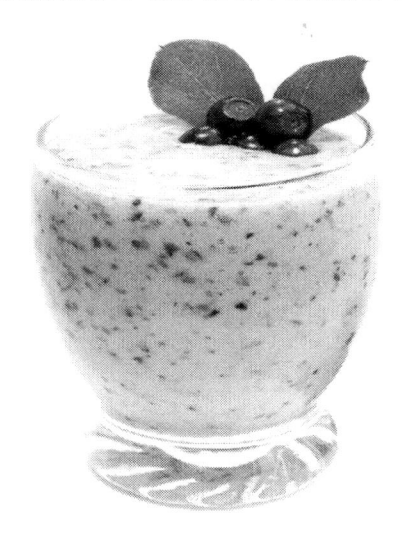

1 cup of blueberries

½ apple (seeded and sliced)

2 oranges peeled and sliced

1 ginger toe peeled

½ cup almond milk

1 cup romaine lettuce or 3-4 stalks

1 cup of ice

Mix all ingredients in a vita mixer or a blender and serve. This makes 2 small glasses. If this is too thick you can add more almond milk or water.

PEAR SMOOTHIE

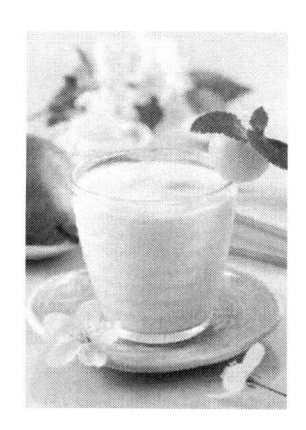

1 pear sliced and seeded

1 orange peeled and cut into quarters

1 ginger toe peeled

½ frozen banana

3-4 stalks of romaine lettuce

1/2 cup celery

1 cup of almond milk

1 cup of ice

Mix all ingredients in a vita mixer or blender and serve. This makes 2 small glasses.

GREEN NECTARINE

5-6 romaine stalks

1/8 cup of aloe vera juice

1 cup spinach

3 nectarines with the seed taken out

2 dates pitted

Splash of lime juice

1 cup of ice

1 cup of almond milk

Mix all ingredients in a vita mixer or blender and serve. This makes 2 small glasses.

BLACKBERRY DREAM

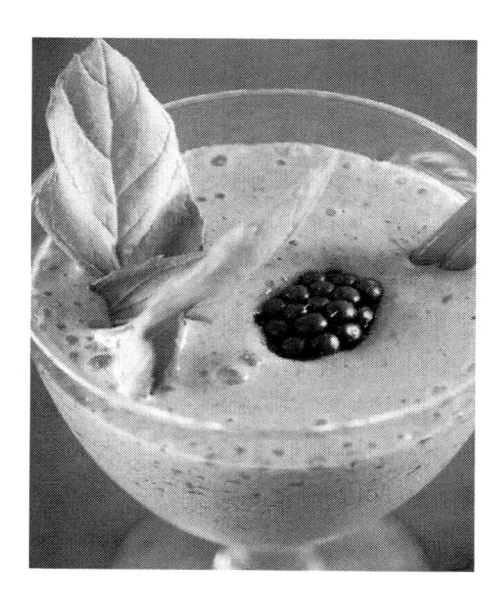

1 raw coconut (scoop out the inside of it)

1 cup frozen blackberries

2 dates pitted

4-5 romaine stalks

½ frozen banana

1 cup almond milk

1 cup of ice

Mix all ingredients in a vita mixer or blender and serve. This makes 2 medium glasses.

MIXED GREEN BERRY

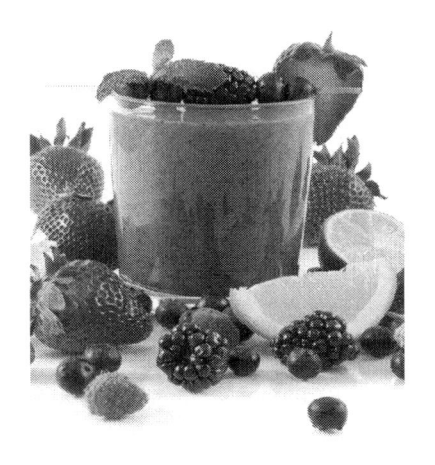

2 cups frozen mixed berries

3 cups of spinach

½ frozen banana

1 cup almond milk

1 cup of ice

1/8 cup of lime juice

1 toe of ginger peeled

Mix all ingredients in a vita mixer or blender and serve. This makes two medium glasses.

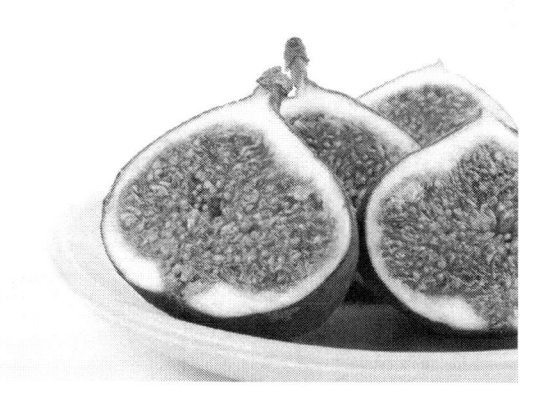

FIGLISIOUS

½ cup blueberries
3-4 figs
1 date pitted
2 cups of spinach
1 orange peeled and quartered
1 cup almond milk
1 cup of ice

Mix all ingredients in a vita mixer or blender and serve.
This makes 2 small glasses.

Raw Appetizers

SPICY SUN DRIED TOMATO & PALANO DIP

TOMATO & AVACADO TOWER

TROPICAL PLAINTAIN SLAW

CILANTRO PESTO DIP

MARIANATED MUSHROOMS

TOMATO, ONION, AND PARM CAPRESE

MANGO SALSA

VEGGIE TORTE

MUSHROOM PATE

SPICY & CHEESY JICAMA FRIES WITH CREAMY TOMATO SAUCE

STUFFED MINI SWEET RED AND YELLOW PEPPERS

GUACAMOLE

EASY SALSA

- GRAPEFRUIT, BEET, AVOCADO TOWER
- JICAMA SALSA
- SPROUT & NORI WRAP
- CHUNKY COWBOY CORN DIP
- TANGY DILL DIP
- COCONUT CURRY DIP
- VEGGY ANTIPASTI

SPICY SUN DRIED TOMATO & PABLANO DIP

1 dried pablano pepper soaked in a small amount of water
1 cup soaked raw cashews
¼ cup olive oil
1 cup soaked sundried tomatoes (keep the liquid from the soaked tomatoes)
Celtic salt and black pepper

Take the pablono pepper that has been soaked and drained. Take the pablano pepper, the drained cashews, olive oil, the sun dried tomatoes, and salt and pepper and put all of the ingredients in a vita mixer and blend until smooth. You will need to add some of the water back into the mixer until it blends smoothly. It just depends on how smooth you like the dip. Then use romaine leaves, carrots, cucumbers to dip.

TOMATO & AVACADO TOWER

3 Small orange tomatoes
3 Small Red Tomatoes
2 Avocados
Olive Oil
Balsamic Vinegar

First take both types of tomatoes and chop into small pieces. Next take the avocados and scoop out the insides and chop into small pieces. Next take the avocado and place in a round area on your presentation plate. Then take the other tomatoes and layer them on the avocado in the shape of a tower. Now drizzle with olive oil and balsamic vinegar. Use the salt and pepper to your taste.

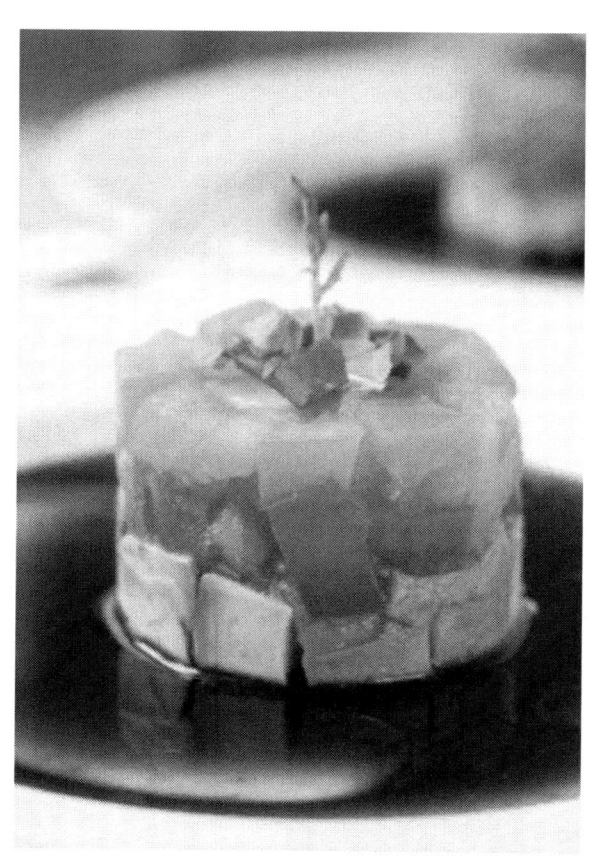

TROPICAL PLANTAIN SLAW

1 head of Napa cabbage shredded thinly
1 red pepper sliced thin
Sauce
1 really ripe plantain
1 orange peeled
½ cup almond butter
¼ cup of olive oil
¼ teaspoon of red pepper flakes
Celtic sea salt and black pepper to taste

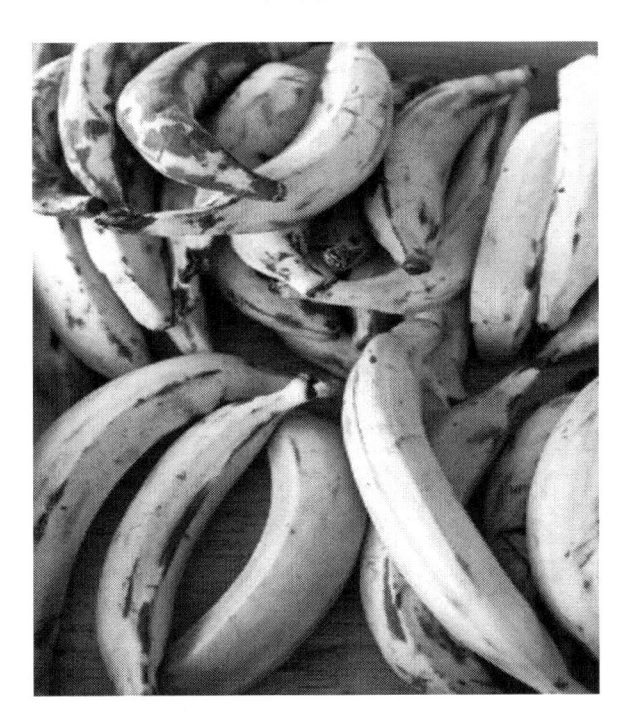

Take the shredded cabbage and thinly sliced red peppers and put in a large bowl. Next take the ingredients for the sauce and blend in a vita mixer until smooth with a medium consistency and then pour the sauce on the cabbage and red peppers and mix well. You can use this slaw for a filling in collard greens, large romaine leaves, or just by itself.

CILANTRO PESTO DIP

1 cup cilantro
½ cup olive oil
2 tablespoon hemp oil
1 cup of pumpkin seeds soaked
Celtic sea salt and black pepper

Mix all ingredients in a vita mixer until smooth. You may want to save some of the water from the pumpkin seeds that were soaking to use to smooth out the dip. The consistency should be a medium consistency. You can use this pesto to dip your veggies in or as a base for your wraps. Either way this is a yummy dip!

MARINATED MUSHROOMS

3 cups of sliced mushrooms of every variety that you like (portabella and crimini work well)
1/8 cup of olive oil
1 tablespoon of vinegar of your choice
1 teaspoon of agave nectar
1 teaspoon of Braggs
Celtic sea salt and black pepper
1 clove of garlic diced small
1 teaspoon of cumin

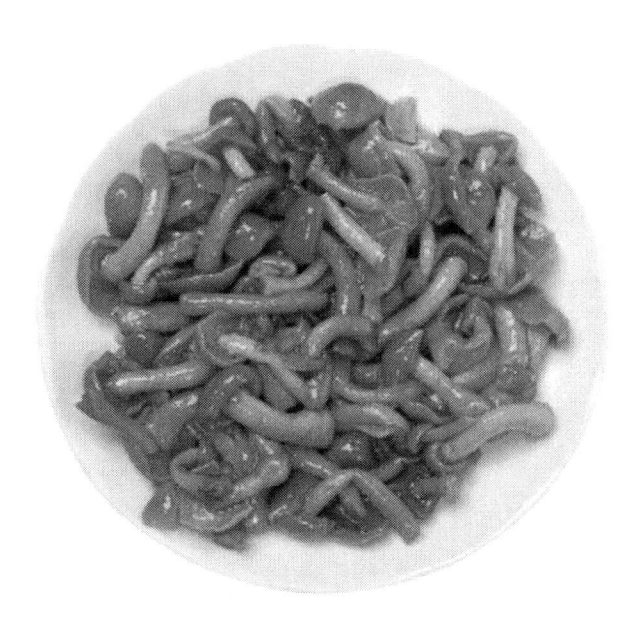

Take all of the liquid ingredients and marinate the mushrooms in the sauce overnight. Then you can use these mushrooms for dipping in sauces, raw pizzas, or just by themselves!

TOMATO, ONION & PARM CAPRESE

1-2 large tomatoes
1 sweet onion
Olive oil and balsamic for the top
¼ cup chopped basil
Parm
½ cup cashews
½ cup pine nuts
1 clove of garlic
½ teaspoon of Braggs
3 tablespoons of nutritional yeast
2 tablespoons of lemon juice
Celtic sea salt

Take and slice the tomatoes and onions in rounds. Next take the pine nuts, cashews, nutritional yeast, garlic, lemon juice, salt, and Braggs and mix in a vita mixer until the mixture is fine. Take the sliced tomatoes and sliced onions and tower them on top of each other and sprinkle them with the parmesan and sprinkle with olive oil, balsamic, and basil.

MANGO SALSA

1 large mango peeled and sliced into small pieces
2 limes
1 cup of cilantro
1 hass avocado diced
1 small jalapeño
1 teaspoon of olive oil
½ red peppers
Celtic salt and black pepper

Take the mango and mix in the juice of the limes, chopped cilantro, diced avocado, jalapeño diced small, and diced red pepper and mix together with 1 teaspoon of olive oil and salt and pepper. Use this for a dip with raw crackers or as a sauce in wraps.

VEGETABLE TORTE

2 green zucchini
2 yellow zucchini

1 cup marinated mushrooms (from this section)
Raw ricotta
1 cup macadamia nuts soaked (save the soaked water)
3 tablespoons of nutritional yeast
$\frac{1}{4}$ cup lemon juice
Celtic sea salt and black pepper to taste

Blend the macadamia nuts with the lemon juice and enough water to make the mixture smooth, and then add the nutritional yeast, salt and pepper.

Take the zucchini's and slice very thin and alternate between marinated mushrooms and ricotta and the zucchini slices until all of the ingredients are gone. Then let set in the refrigerator for 1 hour and then serve with raw crackers or by it!
Thai noodles

2 young coconuts
$\frac{1}{2}$ cup of almond butter
1 lime
1 small banana
1 teaspoon yellow curry (if you want green or red is fine also; it depends on your taste)

½ cup of cilantro
¼ cup Thai basil
1-2 Thai peppers

Take the young coconuts and scoop the young coconut out and be sure to be careful to not break it up too much. Then take the coconut and slice it thinly so that it looks like noodles. In another bowl take the ½ cup of the coconut water, small banana, almond butter, juice of the lime, curry, and salt and pepper and mix until smooth. Take this sauce and pour it over the coconut noodles and then garnish with basil, cilantro, and sliced Thai peppers (it depends on how hot you like it so use accordingly) yum.

MUSHROOM PATE

1 cup of almonds that have been soaked
1 cup of raw sunflower seeds soaked
2 tablespoons of lemon juice
1 red pepper rough chopped
1 carrot chopped
1 cup cilantro
1 clove of garlic
¼ onion chopped
¼ cup nutritional yeast

1 cup of marinated mushrooms
1 tablespoon of Braggs

Take all of the ingredients and mix in a food processor until well mixed and put the ingredients in a glass dish and refrigerate for an hour or so until firm and then serve with raw crackers or veggies.

SPICY & CHEESY JICAMA FRIES WITH CREAMY TOMATO SAUCE

2 large jicama peeled and sliced in the shape of french fries.
$\frac{1}{4}$ teaspoon of cayenne
1 teaspoon of paprika
Salt and pepper
1 tablespoon of lime juice
1 teaspoon of olive oil
2 tablespoons of nutritional yeast

Sauce
$\frac{1}{2}$ cup of raw cashews soaked
3 small roma tomatoes
1/8 cup of olive oil
1 tablespoon of maple syrup
Salt and pepper to taste

Take the sliced jicama and toss with spices and olive oil. Next take the sauce ingredients and mix in a vita mixer until thick like the consistency of ketchup. Now dip the jicama in the sauce and enjoy!

STUFFED MINI SWEET PEPPERS

8-10 mini red and yellow sweet peppers
1 cup of walnuts soaked
½ cup cilantro
Salt and pepper
2 tablespoons of nutritional yeast
1 carrot chopped
1 teaspoon of cumin
½ teaspoon of cayenne
1 tablespoon of lemon juice

Take everything but the red peppers and mix in the vita mixer and blend until mixed well. Take the sweet peppers and cut the tops off and fill them with the mixture and serve.

GUACAMOLE

3 Hass Avocados
¼ Cup Lime Juice
½ Cup diced tomatoes
1 Jalapeño
1 Clove of Garlic
1 Bunch of Cilantro
Salt and Pepper
1 teaspoon of cumin
½ teaspoon of cayenne

Scoop the avocado out of the shells. Next cut the jalapeño in half and take the seeds out. In a vita mixer take the rest of the ingredients except for the tomatoes and blend until smooth. Now add the chopped tomatoes and your ready for your raw burritos.

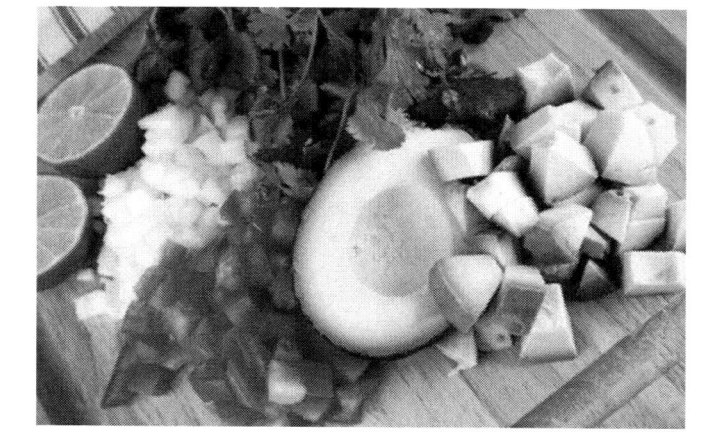

EASY SALSA

5 Tomatoes
½ Cup lime juice
1 Jalapeño
1 bunch of cilantro
½ small onion
1 clove of garlic
Salt and pepper
1 teaspoon of cumin
½ teaspoon of cayenne
1 cup chopped avocado

First take the jalapeño and cut in half and take the seeds out. Then take the rest of the ingredients except for the avocado and blend until choppy with a vita mixer. Now take the chopped avocados and mix them with the ingredients and serve with your favorite raw crackers!

GRAPEFRUIT, AVACADO, & BEET TOWER

2 Grapefruits
2 Avocados
2 beets

Small zucchini flowers
Micro greens
Salt and Pepper
Balsamic vinegar
Olive oil

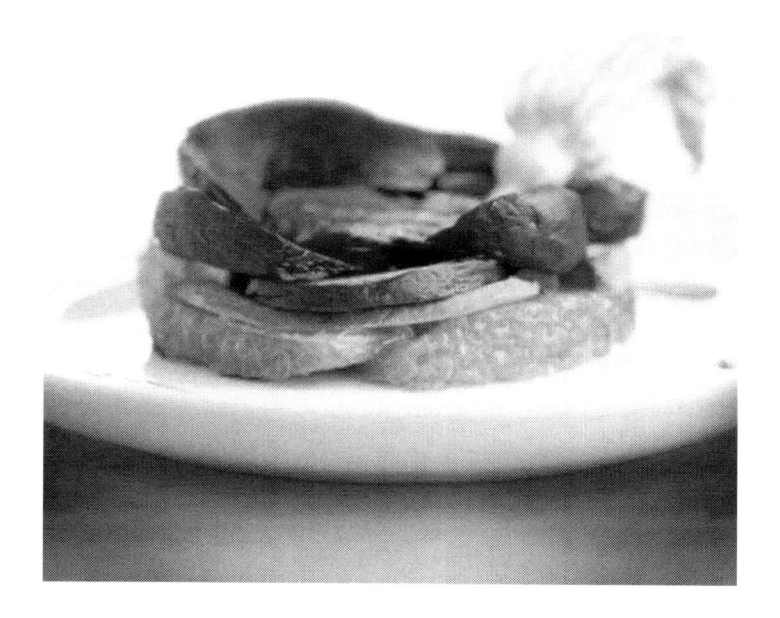

First take the grapefruit and peel them and then slice them in a round circle. Next take the avocados and scoop them out and chop them in small pieces. For the final phase of the tower take the two beets and peel them and slice them really thin and marinate them in with a little orange juice and Braggs for a couple of hours.

Take one round grapefruit slice and add some of the avocado to the top and then a thin slice of the beet. Top with micro greens and zucchini flowers and drizzle with olive oil and balsamic vinegar. Keep doing this until all the ingredients are used up for the towers and serve.

JICAMA SALSA

1 Large Jicama
1 Red Pepper
1 Yellow Pepper
1 Orange
½ Cup Chopped Cilantro
Salt and Pepper

Take the jicama and peel it and chop into small pieces. Next take the peppers and take the seeds out and chop them also into small pieces. Mix the jicama and peppers in a bowl and squeeze the juice of the orange onto the mixture. Now top with the cilantro and serve with dehydrated chips.

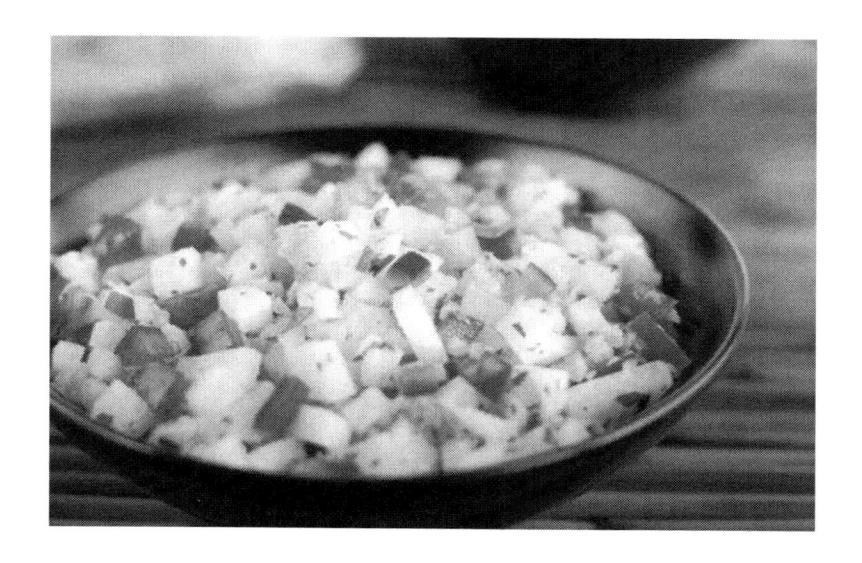

SPROUT & NORI WRAPS

Couple of large handfuls of sunflower sprouts
3 Nori Sheets
Nama Shoyu (raw soy sauce) for dipping

These are so simple and easy! First take the sunflower sprouts (or any sprouts that you prefer) and lay them in the nori sheets and wrap them up tight. Next slice them and place on a plate with the nama shoyu as a dipping sauce. You can use whatever sauce you like. Sometimes I will use an almond butter sauce made with a little almond butter and lime juice.

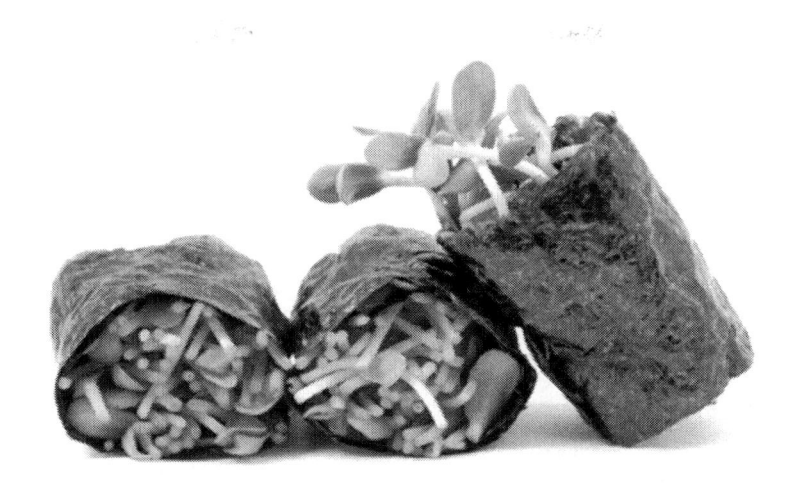

CHUNKY COWBOY CORN DIP

3 Ears of Corn
2 Tablespoons of Hemp Seeds
1 Large Red Pepper
½ Cup of Cilantro
Salt and Pepper to Taste
2 Tablespoons of lime juice
½ Teaspoon of cumin

First take the ears of corn and slice the corn off of the cob. Next take the red pepper and cut into small pieces. Mix the corn, red pepper, lime juice, s

& p, cumin, and sprinkle with hemp seeds. You can eat this as a side salad or dip with raw crackers.

TANGY DILL DIP

1 Bunch of fresh dill
1 Cup of Cashews (soaked)
¼ cup of olive oil
1 Clove of garlic
2 Tablespoons of lime juice
½ teaspoon of sage
½ teaspoon of thyme
Salt & pepper

Take the soaked cashews and drain (save the liquid in case you may need it for a thinner sauce) and put in a vita mixer along with the rest of the ingredients and blend until smooth. Use on wraps or as a dip with raw chips.

COCONUT CURRY CARROT DIP

4 Medium carrots
1 Cup Macadamia nuts (soaked)
1 teaspoon curry powder

2 Tablespoons of coconut water
Basil for garnish
Salt and Pepper

Take the carrots and clean and peel them and put them in a vita mixer along with the rest of the ingredients until smooth. Garnish with the basil and serve.

VEGGY ANITPASTI

1 Cup of Marinated Portobello's
1 Small Eggplant
1 Red Pepper
½ Bunch of Asparagus
½ cup of balsamic vinegar
½-3/4 Cup of olive oil
2 small zucchini
Salt and Pepper

First take the eggplant and zucchini and slice with a mandolin (or very fine). Then slice the red pepper thinly and trim the asparagus. Now take the above ingredients and soak for 1 hour in the balsamic vinegar and olive oil. Drain and place nicely on a platter with raw chips and serve.

Raw Soups

Creamy Avocado and Cucumber Medley

Macho Gazpacho

Creamy Red Pepper Soup

Creamy Pea Soup

Creamy Carrot Fennel Soup

Thai Coconut Lemon grass Soup

Spicy Watermelon Tomato Soup

Creamy Celery and Green Apple Soup

Raw Creamy Celery Soup

Raw Tomato Soup

Sun Dried Tomato and Pablano Chili Soup

Creamy Butternut Squash Soup

Spinach Soup

Sweet Summer Watermelon Soup

Mango/Madness

Peanut Soup

Black Pepper and Zucchini Soup

Coconut and Macadamia Nut Soup

Summer Romaine Soup

Kale Nutrition Soup

Creamy Avocado and Cucumber Medley

4 large organic cucumbers, peeled
4 organic celery stalks
2 Hass avocados peeled and pitted
2 limes
4 cups purified water

Put all the ingredients in the Vita-Mixer and chill and serve garnished with cilantro sprigs! Yum!

Macho Gazpacho

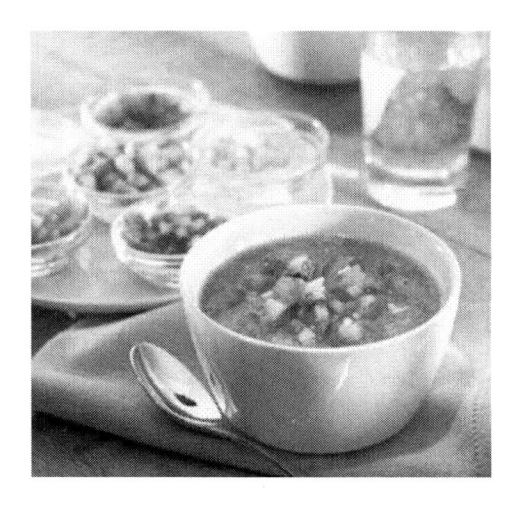

4 cups Roma tomatoes
1 cup diced and seeded tomatoes

1 CUP PEELED, SEEDED CUCUMBER DICED
2 CUP RED, GREEN, AND YELLOW PEPPERS
2 LIMES SQUEEZED INTO SOUP
2 AVOCADOS CUT INTO SMALL PIECES
3 CLOVES OF GARLIC CRUSHED
1 SMALL BUNCH OF CILANTRO CHOPPED
1 SMALL JALAPENO, SEEDED AND MINCED
1/2 GREEN ONION MINCED
1 TEASPOON SEA SALT
FRESH GROUND BLACK PEPPER

PUREE THE 4 CUPS OF ROMA TOMATOES AND THEN ADD ALL THE OTHER INGREDIENTS AND VOILA' YOU HAVE MACHO GAZPACHO!

Creamy Red Pepper Soup

3 ORGANIC RED BELL PEPPERS SEEDED AND STEMS REMOVED
1 YOUNG COCONUT
2 CLOVES OF GARLIC
3 TABLESPOONS COLD PRESSED EXTRA VIRGIN OLIVE OIL
1 BUNCH OF ORGANIC CILANTRO
2 TEASPOONS OF SEA SALT
2 LIMES SQUEEZED

If you like it spicier you can add a jalapeno or some cayenne pepper it just depends on how hot you like it.

Use all the coconut meat and juice. Then mix all the ingredients in a Vita-Mixer except half of the cilantro (use the rest as a garnish) and you have red pepper soup. This is a great soup for boosting your vitamin C intake so eat up!

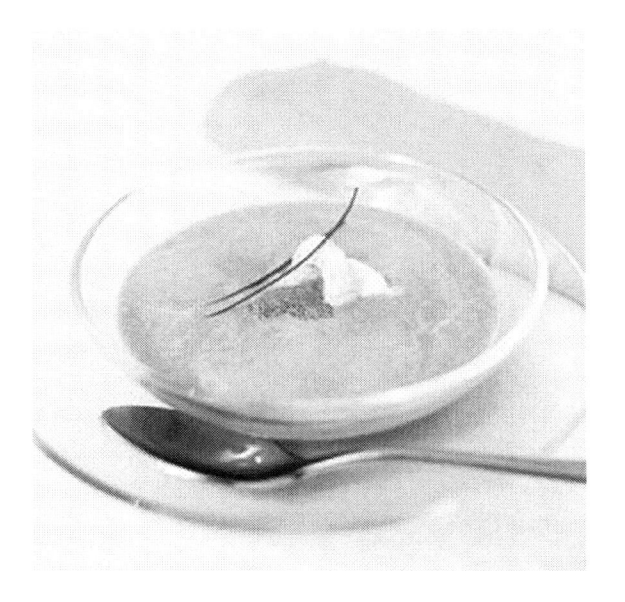

Creamy Pea Soup

2 cups organic fresh peas

2 CUPS OF PURIFIED WATER
1 LARGE RIPE AVOCADO
1 BUNCH BASIL LEAVES
3 CLOVES OF ORGANIC GARLIC
1 TEASPOON OF SEA SALT

BLEND ALL INGREDIENTS IN A VITA MIXER AND BLEND UNTIL SMOOTH!

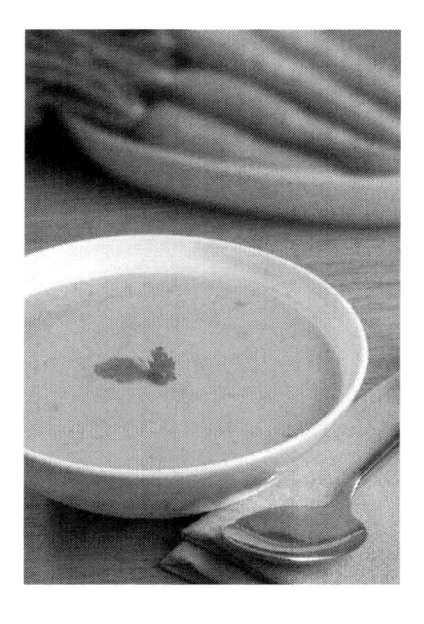

CREAMY CARROT FENNEL SOUP

4 CUPS OF PURIFIED WATER

4 ORGANIC CARROTS

1 LARGE AVOCADO

1 ORGANIC APPLE OF YOUR CHOICE

1 LARGE FENNEL BULB CHOPPED

1 TEASPOON OF SEA SALT

2 TABLESPOONS OF DILL WEED

BLEND ALL INGREDIENTS IN A VITA-MIXER UNTIL CREAMY AND ENJOY!

THAI COCONUT LEMON GRASS SOUP

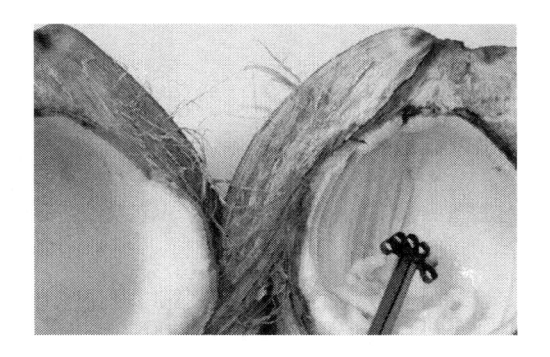

2 CUPS YOUNG COCONUT MEAT

2 CUPS COCONUT WATER

3 TABLESPOONS OF GINGER

1 TABLESPOON THAI CHILI PASTE

2 CLOVES OF GARLIC

1 BUNCH OF ORGANIC CILANTRO

2 TABLESPOON OF GROUND LEMON GRASS
1/2 BUNCH OF ITALIAN PARSLEY
3 TABLESPOONS OF COLD PRESSED OLIVE OIL
3 TABLESPOONS TAMARI
SEA SALT TO YOUR TASTING

BLEND ALL INGREDIENTS IN THE VITA-MIXER AND THERE YOU HAVE A GREAT HEALTHY MEAL!

Spicy Watermelon Tomato Soup

4 CUPS WATERMELON SEEDED
2 CUPS ANY KIND OF TOMATOES
1 CUP DICED TOMATOES
1 CUP DICED PEELED CUCUMBER
1 CUP DICED GREEN AND RED PEPPERS
1/4-1/2 (DEPENDING ON YOUR TASTES I LIKE A LOT OF LIME) CUP KEY LIME JUICE
1 LARGE JALAPEÑO DICED INTO SMALL PIECES
1 LARGE BUNCH OF CILANTRO CHOPPED FINE
1 LARGE PIECE OF GINGER PEELED
SALT AND PEPPER TO TASTE

FIRST PUREE THE 4 CUPS OF WATERMELON AND 2 CUPS OF TOMATOES ALONG WITH THE GINGER IN A VITA-MIXER. THEN ADD ALL THE OTHER DICED INGREDIENTS AND EAT UP! THIS IS GREAT FOR summer or really anytime. It is very refreshing chilled!

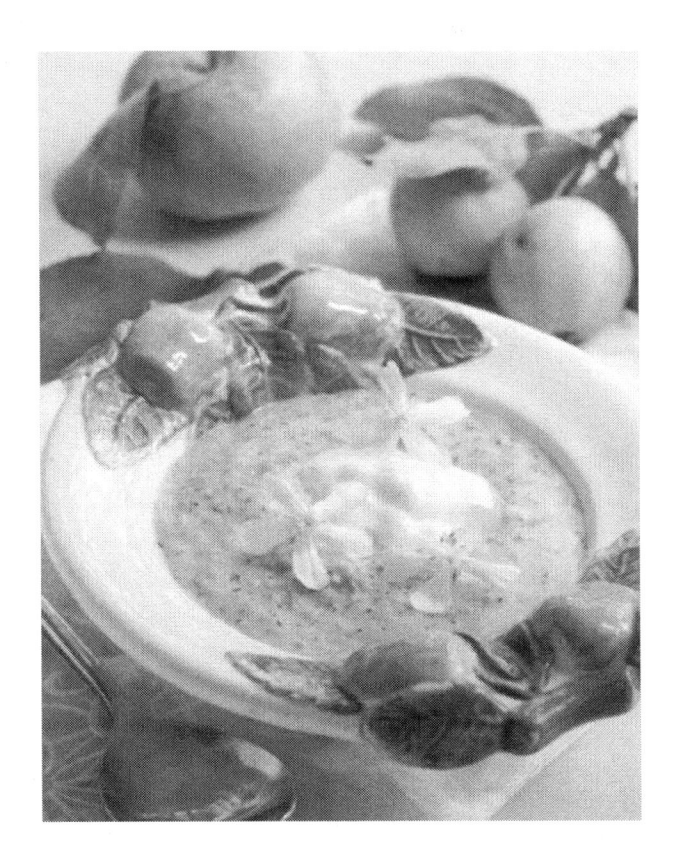

Creamy Celery and Green Apple Soup

1 bunch organic celery
4 large organic granny smith apples
1/4 -1/2 cup lemon juice (depends on your taste)
1/4 cup cold pressed olive oil

2 tablespoons of coconut butter (this you can find at most health food stores)
2 cups soaked raw macadamia nuts (soak for at least 2 hours)
1 cup water or to your thickness
See salt and black pepper to taste
You can add chopped parsley for a garnish or even both red and green apples mixed to give it a nice color.
This is a bit of a labor of love soup but it is very tasty! First cut the celery into small pieces and only 3 of the granny smith apples and put into the vita mixer.

Once this is done drain the juice from the pulp and save both. Now wash the soaked macadamia nuts and throw them in the vita mixer along with the strained juice, water, olive oil, lemon juice, and s & p if you want a thicker soup you can add back some of the pulp. Now that this is done you garnish with the last granny smith apple that you cut into small bites size pieces and serve. You can add white truffle oil for an even richer soup or if you are having quests due to the price of the oil.

Raw Creamy Celery Soup

    1 bunch of celery
    1/2 cup olive oil
    1/4 cup lemon juice
    4 cups of water
    2 teaspoons of agave nectar
    1 cup soaked raw cashews
    3/4 cup of parsley

You can also top this soup off with chopped avocado, sliced carrots, or chopped red pepper and parsley.

Blend all ingredients in a Vita Mixer until smooth and creamy. If you want the soup thicker just use 1 cup less water in the recipe. This is great soup for the summer chilled or right out of the Vita Mixer!

Raw Tomato Soup

    8 large tomatoes
    2 cloves of garlic peeled
    $\frac{1}{4}$ cup of lime juice
    1/8 cup of olive oil
    Salt and pepper to your liking

Tablespoon of chopped basil

Tablespoon of chopped oregano

This is one of the easiest raw soups to make! Just blend all ingredients with a Vita Mixer until smooth consistency and garnish with a few basil sprigs!

Sun Dried Tomato and Poblano Chili Soup (this is a hot one)

1 cup of sun dried tomatoes soaked for 4-5 hours

2-3 dried poblanos soaked for 4-5 hours

3 cups of water

½ cup of lemon juice

¼ cup of olive oil

1 small peeled cucumber

Chopped parsley

Chopped cilantro

Salt and pepper to taste

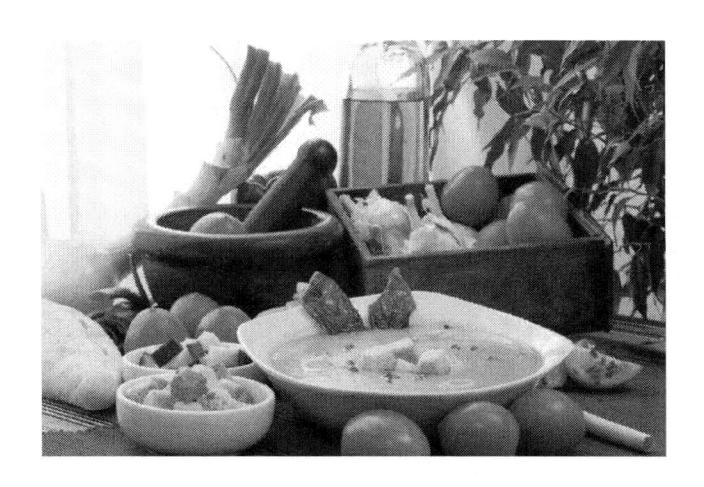

Rinse the soaked tomatoes and poblano chilies and put them along with the rest of the ingredients in the Vita Mixer and garnish with cilantro and extra slice of lemons or limes!

Creamy Butternut Squash Soup

> 3 cups peeled and cut into smaller pieces for the Vita Mixer
> 1/8 cup olive oil
> 1/8 cup of raw peanut butter
> 2 tablespoons of parsley
> 1 teaspoon of curry powder
> ¼ lime juice
> ¾ cup of water

Sea salt of Braggs to your liking
1 tablespoon of agave nectar

Mix all of the above ingredients into a Vita Mixer until smooth and garnish with fresh parsley sprigs!

Spinach Soup

1 cup of almond milk
1 cup of water
5 cups of spinach
2 small cucumbers peeled
1 clove of garlic
¼ cup of almond butter
1/8 cup of lime juice
1/8 cup of hemp oil
Salt and pepper to taste or Braggs if you like

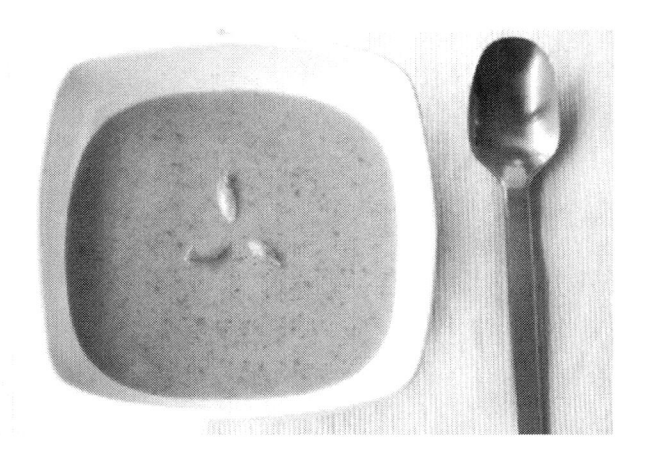

Mix all ingredients in the Vita Mixer and garnish with a few slices of cucumber!

Sweet Summer Watermelon Soup

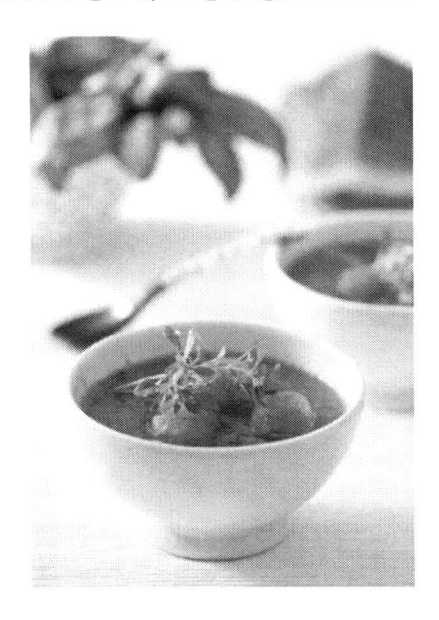

6 cups of watermelon
1 cup honey dew melon
1 cup of ice
½ cup of pineapple juice
Chopped mint

Mix all ingredients in a Vita Mixer except 1 cup of the watermelon (cut into small chunks and use as a garnish)! This

IS A GREAT SOUP TO COOL YOU OFF IN THE SUMMER!

Mango Madness

4 LARGE RIPE MANGOES PEELED AND CUT INTO PIECES (JUST SO THAT THE MANGO FLESH IS SEPARATED FROM THE SEED)
$\frac{1}{4}$ CUP LIME JUICE
2 CUP ORANGE JUICE
3 PITTED DATES
CHOPPED MINT

MIX ALL INGREDIENTS EXCEPT ONE OF THE MANGOES (SAVE IT FOR GARNISH IN THE SOUP) IN A VITA MIXER AND GARNISH WITH THE EXTRA MANGO AND CHOPPED MINT!

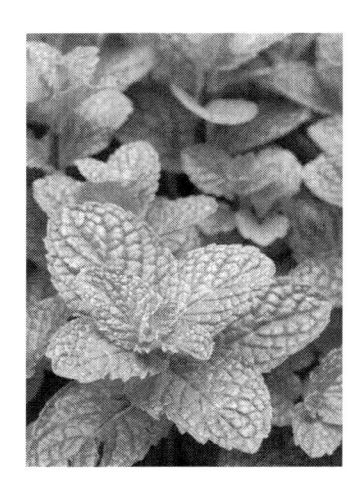

PEANUT SOUP

    2 CUPS WATER
    1 CUP ORANGE JUICE
    2 RIPE BANANAS
    1 TEASPOON CURRY POWDER
    1 CUP NATURAL PEANUT BUTTER
    $\frac{1}{4}$ CUP LIME JUICE
    1 TABLESPOON PEELED GINGER ROOT
    1 CLOVE OF GARLIC
    CHOPPED CILANTRO

MIX ALL INGREDIENTS EXCEPT THE CILANTRO IN A VITA MIXER AND BLEND UNTIL SMOOTH. GARNISH WITH CHOPPED PEANUTS AND CHOPPED CILANTRO! YUM!

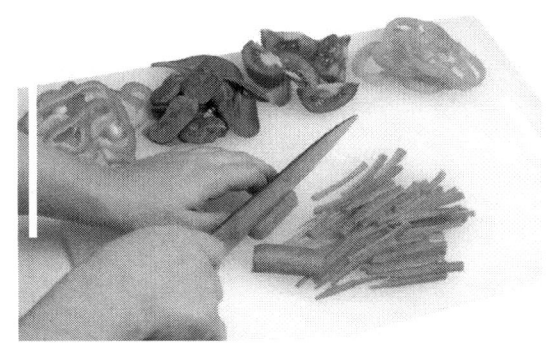

BLACK PEPPER AND ZUCCHINI SOUP

    4 PEELED ZUCCHINIS
    4 STALKS OF CELERY

2 CUPS OF WATER
¼ CUP OF OLIVE OIL
1 TABLESPOON OF BLACK PEPPER
1 CLOVE OF GARLIC
SALT TO TASTE

BLEND ALL INGREDIENTS IN A VITA MIXER AND GARNISH WITH MORE BLACK PEPPER! SPICY BUT GOOD!

COCONUT AND MACADAMIA NUT SOUP

2 CUPS RAW MACADAMIA NUTS SOAKED FOR SEVERAL HOURS
1 RAW COCONUT SCOOPED AND THE WATER SAVED
2 CUPS EXTRA COCONUT WATER
¼ LIME JUICE
1/8 CUP OF MACADAMIA NUT OIL
SALT AND PEPPER TO TASTE
CILANTRO FOR GARNISH

DRAIN THE SOAKED MACADAMIA NUTS AND PUT THE REST OF THE INGREDIENTS IN THE VITA MIXER AND BLEND UNTIL SMOOTH. GARNISH WITH CHOPPED MACADAMIA NUTS, RAW SHREDDED COCONUT, AND CILANTRO! YUM YOU

WILL HAVE MORE FRIENDS THAN YOU WANT WITH THIS SOUP!

Summer Romaine Soup

1 head of romaine lettuce
2 stalks of celery
1 small peeled cucumber
1 cup of water
¼ cup lemon juice
1 small piece of ginger peeled
Salt and pepper to taste
Garnish with chopped cilantro

Blend all ingredients in a Vita Mixer and blend until smooth. Garnish with chopped cilantro! This is a nice a refreshing summer soup!

Kale Nutrition Soup

6 cups of kale
2 cups of water
1 peeled cucumber
¼ cup of lemon juice
1/8 cup of olive oil

½ CUP OF FLAT LEAF PARSLEY
3 CELERY STALKS
SALT AND PEPPER TO TASTE

MIX ALL INGREDIENTS TOGETHER IN A VITA MIXER AND BLEND UNTIL SMOOTH. THE CONSISTENCY WILL BE A LITTLE ON THE THICKER SIDE AND GARNISH WITH CHOPPED CUCUMBERS! THIS IS DELISH AND NUTRISH!

Salads and Dressings

Endive salad with lemon dressing

Rainbow Kale Salad

Tropical Arugula Salad

Fennel, Avocado, & apple Salad

Raspberry & hazelnut salad

Wakame salad

strawberry, walnut, & spinach salad

Tropical Fruit Salad

Pear and Arugula Salad

cucumber salad

Greek salad with tahini dressing

beet and carrot salad

summer watermelon & cucumber salad

Green pea & Mint salad

Rawsparagus salad

Sweet Potato & Avocado Salad

Sesame Garlic Broccoli Salad

Zucchini Dill Salad

Red Cabbage and Beet Salad

Shaved Parsnip and Cherry Salad

Endive Salad with Lemon Dressing

5 small endives cleaned and sliced into bite size pieces
1 red pepper chopped small
Dressing
4 tablespoons of olive oil
3 tablespoons of lemon juice
1 tablespoon of cilantro
Salt and pepper to taste

Chop the endive and red pepper and toss with the dressing and serve!

Avocado & Butter Lettuce Salad

1 head of butter lettuce
2 Hass avocado
1 tablespoon hemp seeds
2 tablespoons of lemon infused olive oil
Salt and pepper to taste

Wash the butter lettuce and spin dry. Take and cut the lettuce into bite sized pieces toss with the avocado sliced into small pieces. Next take the lemon olive oil and drizzle it on the top of the salad and sprinkle with hemp seeds! Yum this is a quick and easy salad that has lots of flavor!

Rainbow Kale Salad with Creamy Dressing

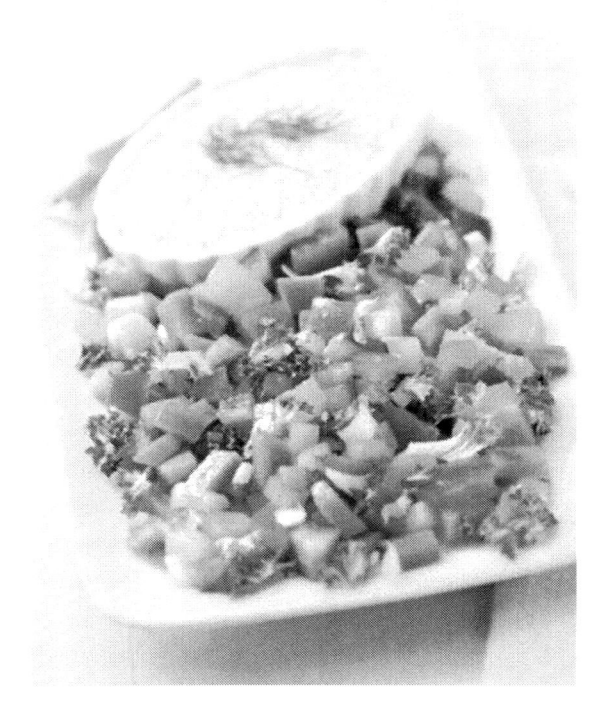

1 bundle of kale
1 Red pepper
1 Green Pepper
1 Yellow pepper

DRESSING
½ CUP CASHEWS SOAKED
½ CUP OLIVE OIL
¼ CUP OF LEMON JUICE
SALT AND PEPPER

FIRST TAKE AND CHOPPED THE KALE INTO BITE SIZE PIECES. NEXT TAKE THE PEPPERS AND CUT IN HALF AND TAKE THE SEEDS OUT AND THEN CHOPPED INTO SMALL PIECES.
FOR THE DRESSING TAKE THE SOAKED CASHEWS (DRAINED), OLIVE OIL, LEMON JUICE, AND SALT AND PEPPER AND BLEND UNTIL SMOOTH.
NOW TAKE THE DRESSING AND TOSS WITH ALL OF THE VEGGIES OR PUT THE DRESSING ON THE SIDE AND SERVE.

TROPICAL ARUGULA SALAD

6 CUPS OF ARUGULA OR ROCKET
1 PALMA GRANITE (PEELED AND THE SEEDS TAKEN OUT)
2 ORANGE
1 GRAPEFRUIT
1 TABLESPOON OF AGAVE NECTAR
¼ CUP OLIVE OIL
SALT AND PEPPER TO TASTE

First take the grapefruit and 1 orange and peel and cut into smaller pieces. Then take the juice of the last orange and agave nectar and olive oil and whisk together to make the dressing. Now take the dressing and toss in on the arugula and add the orange and grapefruit slices and palm granite pieces and serve. This is a great summer salad or great for brunch on the weekends.

Fennel, Avocado, & Apple Salad

2 Fennel Bulbs
2 Avocados
2 Red Apples
¼ Cup fresh mint
1/8 Cup Olive Oil
¼ Cup Lime Juice
Salt and Pepper

First take the fennel and cut the tops off and take the bulbs and cut into smaller pieces. Next take the avocado and cut in half and scoop the avocado out and cut into bite size pieces. Now take the apples and cut the cores out and slice into smaller bite size pieces. Take all oil, mint and lime juice and whisk together and pour it over the mixture and salt and pepper to taste.

Raspberry and Hazelnut salad

6 cups of baby greens
1 Cup of raw hazelnut
1 ½ cup of raspberries
½ Cup of hazelnut oil
1 Tablespoon of agave nectar
salt and pepper to taste

First take the greens and place in a large bowl. Take ½ cup of raspberries, agave nectar and the olive oil and salt and pepper and mix with a blender to make the dressing. Next take the hazelnuts and chop into small pieces and toss them into the greens. Now toss with the dressing and place the whole raspberries on the top and serve.

Wakame salad

2 cups of wakame cut into strips
2 Tablespoons of rice vinegar (or whichever type you like)
1 Tablespoon of sesame oil
1 teaspoon of agave nectar
1 tablespoon of raw sesame seeds
salt and pepper to taste

First take the cut wakame and soak in a small bowl for 10-20 minutes, then drain. Next take the vinegar, oil, agave nectar, and whisk together and pour over the wakame and sprinkle with sesame seeds.

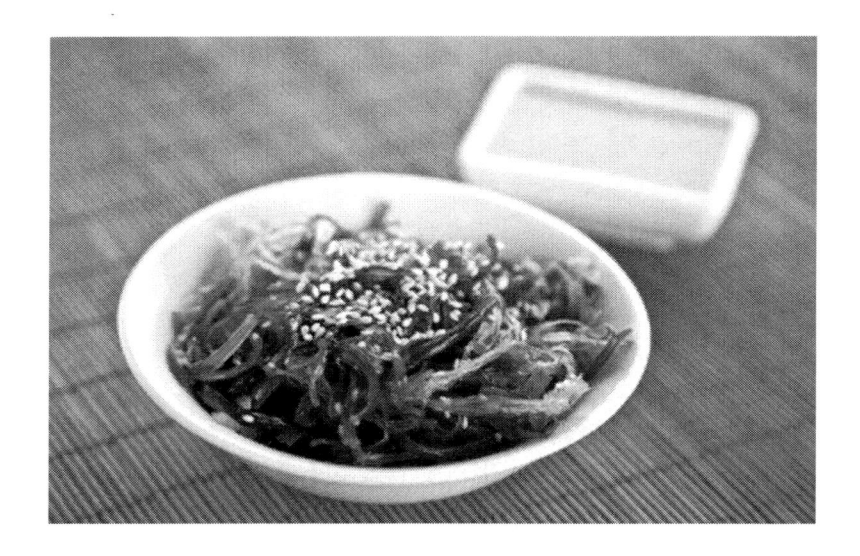

Strawberry & Walnut Spinach Salad

1 quart of fresh strawberries
6-8 cups of fresh spinach
1 cup of raw walnuts chopped
¼ cup balsamic vinegar

½ CUP OF OLIVE OIL
1 TEASPOON OF AGAVE NECTAR
SALT AND PEPPER TO TASTE

First take the spinach and place in a large bowl. Next take the strawberries and slice into thin slices. Take the olive oil, balsamic, and agave nectar and whisk and drizzle over the spinach and add the chopped walnuts and strawberries and toss slightly and serve.

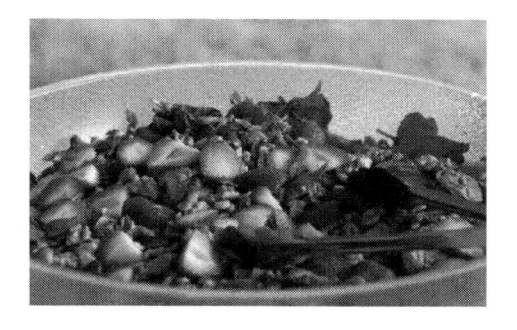

Tropical Fruit salad

3-4 KIWIS
2 ORANGES
1 PINT OF STRAWBERRIES
2-3 PLUMS
1 CUP OF POMEGRANATE SEEDS

First take and peel and slice the kiwis and oranges. Next clean and slice the strawberries. Then slice the plums. Take and mixture and mix in a large bowl and sprinkle with a little lemon juice and a small amount of maple syrup and serve. Great for brunches.

Pear and Arugula Salad

2 Bartlett Pears
5 Cups of Arugula
½ Cup chopped pecans
2 Tablespoons of lemon juice
1 Tablespoon of walnut oil
Salt and Pepper to taste

First take the pear and slice with a mandolin or very fine. Put the arugula, pears, and pecans in a bowl and drizzle with lemon juice, walnut oil, and salt and pepper. Toss & Serve.

Cucumber salad

2 Large English cucumbers
2 Tablespoons of Dill Chopped
1 Tablespoon of agave nectar
¼ Cup cider vinegar
Salt and Pepper to taste
First take the cucumbers and thinly slice lengthwise and toss with the rest of the

INGREDIENTS AND GARNISH WITH MORE DILL. YOU CAN MAKE THIS AHEAD OF TIME SO THAT IT WILL HAVE MORE TIME TO MARINATE.

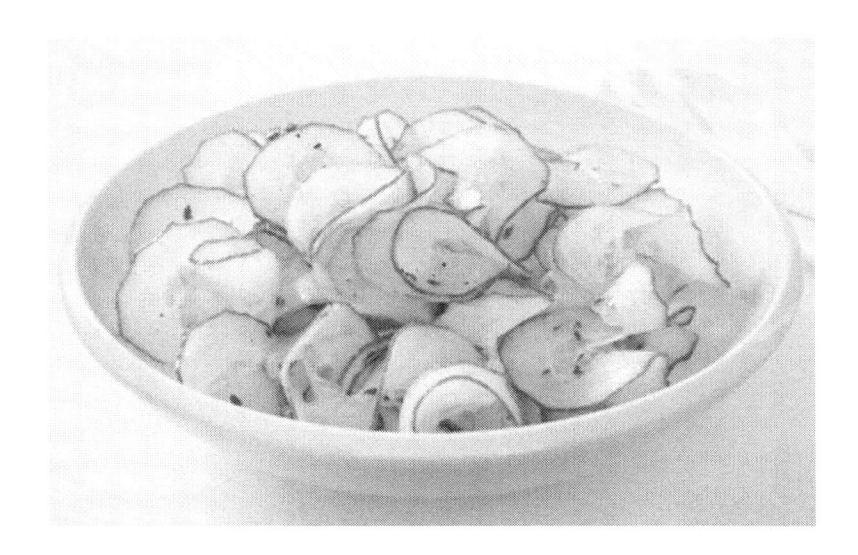

GREEK SALAD WITH TAHINI DRESSING

2 CUCUMBERS
4 TOMATOES
1 GREEN PEPPER
1 SMALL SWEET ONION
DRESSING:

4 tablespoons of Nama Shoyu
2 tablespoons of tahini
2 tablespoons of lemon juice
2 tablespoons of sesame oil
1 tablespoon of agave nectar
1 clove of garlic
Salt and pepper to taste
1 Tablespoon of sesame seeds

First take the cucumbers, tomatoes, and green peppers and cut into small pieces. Next make the dressing with a Vita Mixer and toss on vegetables. Garnish with sesame seeds.

Beet and Carrot Salad

2 beets
3 medium carrots
3 tablespoons of chopped parsley
2 tablespoons of orange juice
1 tablespoon of olive oil
Salt and pepper to taste

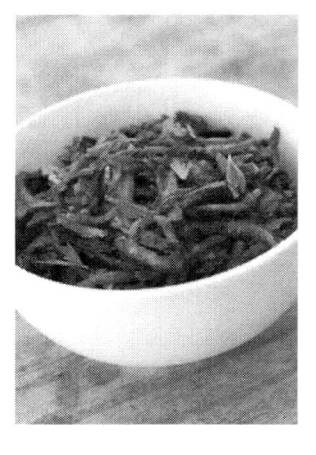

First take the beet and shred into small slivers with a food processor and next do the same with the carrots. Toss the beets and carrots with the orange juice, olive oil, parsley, and salt and pepper. Serve.

Summer Watermelon & Cucumber Salad

4 cups of chopped watermelon
2 cucumbers peeled and chopped
2 tablespoons of raw pine nuts
1 tablespoon of agave nectar
1 tablespoon of lemon juice
1 tablespoon of macadamia oil
$\frac{1}{4}$ cup chopped mint

Take the agave nectar, lemon juice, macadamia oil, and mint and whisk together. Toss the watermelon and cucumber with the dressing and serve.

Pea & Mint Salad

2 cups of fresh peas
1 cup of fresh mint
1 lemon
1 bib lettuce
2 tablespoons of olive oil
2 dates
Salt and pepper to taste

First take the mint, olive oil, dates, juice from the lemon and use a Vita Mixer to make a dressing. Next take the fresh peas and chopped bib lettuce and toss with the dressing and sprinkle with some lemon zest and hemp seeds. This is a great summer salad!

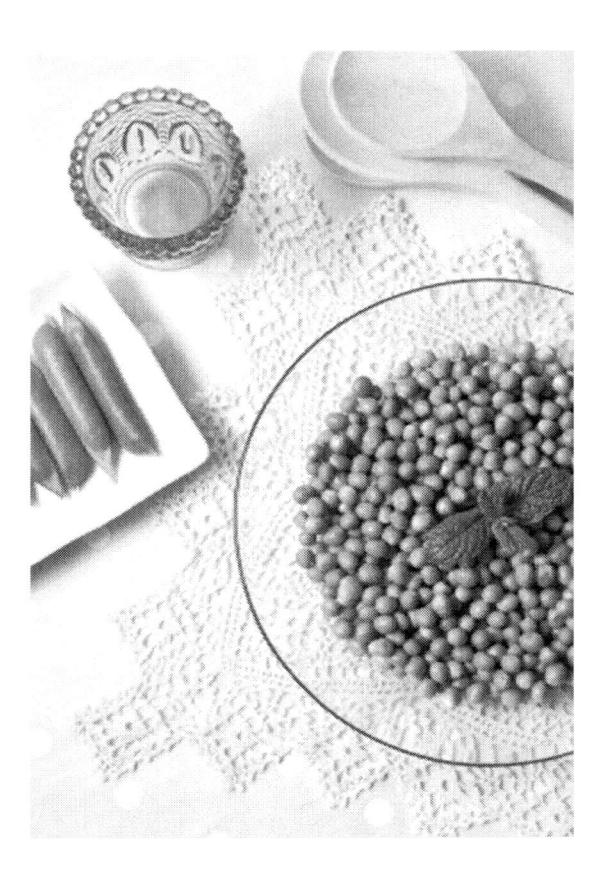

Rawsparagus Salad

1 bunch of asparagus
½ cup of mint
1 tablespoon of basil
¼ cup chopped pecans
1 lemon
2 tablespoon of apple cider vinegar
4 tablespoons of olive oil
salt and pepper to taste

First take the mint, basil, juice of 1 lemon, vinegar, and olive oil and whisk together for the dressing. Next take the asparagus and break the ends off and then cut into 2 inch pieces and then cut them in half and put the dressing on the asparagus and toss and serve.

Sweet Potato & Avocado Salad

2 medium sweet potatoes
1 clove of garlic
2 firm avocados
½ cup chopped raw peanuts
2 tablespoons of apple cider vinegar
4 tablespoons of olive oil
salt and pepper to taste

First take the sweet potatoes and clean and peel them. Next take the sweet potatoes and

GRATE THEM. TAKE THE CLOVE OF GARLIC AND PRESS IT THROUGH A GARLIC PRESS SO THAT IT IS VERY FINE. TAKE THE SWEET POTATOES, GARLIC, APPLE CIDER VINEGAR, OLIVE OIL, AND SALT AND PEPPER AND MIX THOROUGHLY. NOW TAKE THE AVOCADOS AND CUT IN HALF AND TAKE THE SEEDS OUT AND CUT INTO THIN CRESCENT PIECES AND LIGHTLY TOSS THEM WITH THE SWEET POTATOES AND TOP WITH RAW CHOPPED PEANUTS.

SESAME GARLIC BROCCOLI

1 LARGE HEAD OF BROCCOLI
2 CLOVES OF GARLIC
1 TEASPOON OF CUMIN
1 TABLESPOON OF SESAME SEEDS
1 TABLESPOON OF SESAME OIL
1/8 CUP OF OLIVE OIL
2 TABLESPOONS OF OLIVE OIL
RED PEPPER FLAKES TO YOUR TASTE
SALT AND PEPPER

FIRST TAKE THE BROCCOLI AND CUT INTO SMALL FLORETS. NEXT TAKE THE CHOPPED GARLIC, CUMIN, OILS, AND VINEGAR AND MIX IN A VITA MIXER. NEXT TAKE THE DRESSING AND TOSS WITH THE BROCCOLI AND SPRINKLE WITH RED PEPPER FLAKES AND SESAME

SEEDS AND LET MARINATE FOR AT LEAST ONE HOUR OR DEPENDING UPON YOUR TASTE BUDS.

ZUCCHINI AND DILL SALAD

2 SMALL GREEN ZUCCHINI
2 SMALL YELLOW SQUASH
1 CLOVE OF GARLIC
1 SMALL SHALLOT
1 TABLESPOON OF DILL
2 LEMONS (FOR THE JUICE AND THE ZEST)
$\frac{1}{4}$ CUP OF OLIVE OIL
$\frac{1}{4}$ CUP RAW WALNUTS CHOPPED FINE
SALT AND PEPPER TO TASTE

FIRST TAKE THE ZUCCHINI AND SQUASH AND USE A MANDOLIN TO SLICE VERY THIN. NEXT TAKE THE GARLIC, OLIVE OIL, SHALLOT, THE JUICE OF THE LEMONS AND THE ZEST AND USE A VITA MIXER TO MAKE A DRESSING. TOSS THE ZUCCHINI AND SQUASH WITH THE DRESSING AND SPRINKLE WITH THE DILL, CHOPPED WALNUTS, SALT AND PEPPER.

RED CABBAGE SALAD

1/2 HEAD OF RED CABBAGE SHREDDED
2 BEETS PEELED AND SHREDDED
1/8 CUP OF OLIVE OIL
3 TABLESPOON OF NUTRITIONAL YEAST

1 LEMON AND THE ZEST
¼ CUP OF PUMPKIN SEEDS
SALT AND PEPPER

TAKE THE OLIVE OIL, NUTRITIONAL YEAST, THE JUICE OF 1 LEMON, SALT, AND PEPPER AND MIX IN THE VITA MIXER. TOSS THE SHREDDED CABBAGE WITH THE DRESSING AND SPRINKLE WITH THE PUMPKIN SEEDS AND SERVE.

SHAVED PARSNIP AND CHERRY SALAD

1 HEAD OF ROMAINE
1 PARSNIP
½ CUP OF DRIED CHERRIES
1 TABLESPOON OF APPLE CIDER VINEGAR
3 TABLESPOONS OF OLIVE OIL
SALT AND PEPPER TO TASTE

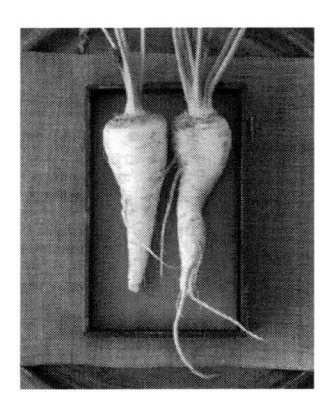

TAKE THE ROMAINE AND SLICE INTO THIN PIECES. NEXT TAKE THE PARSNIP AND PEEL IT AND SLICE IT

INTO THIN LONG PIECES. NEXT TAKE THE OLIVE OIL, VINEGAR, SALT AND PEPPER AND WHISK TOGETHER TO MAKE A DRESSING AND TOSS WITH THE ROMAINE AND PARSNIPS AND TOP WITH THE DRIED CHERRIES.

Raw dinners

Collard Wraps

Crunchy Lettuce Wraps

Sweet Nori Wraps

Veggie Nori Wraps

Sun Dried Tomato & Arugula Pizza

Mushroom & Tomato Pesto Pizza

Mediterranean Burritos

Alfredo Raw Pasta

Pesto Linguini

Spaghetti Squash Pasta & Spicy Garlic Sauce

Italian Caprese Towers

Lasagna

Stuffed Tomatoes

Ravioli

Quinoa Summer Salad

Thai Wild Rice Salad

Sweet Summer Wild Rice Salad

Raw Burger

Lentil Salad

Italian Barley Salad

COLLARD WRAPS

6 medium collard leaves (washed with the stem taken off if they are too long)
1cup shredded carrots
1 cup 1 inch thinly sliced cucumbers
1 cup thinly sliced red peppers
1 cup sprouts
¼ cup raw sunflower seeds
½ cup of some type of spread like raw pesto, raw sundried tomato spread, hummus (whatever one you like the best)

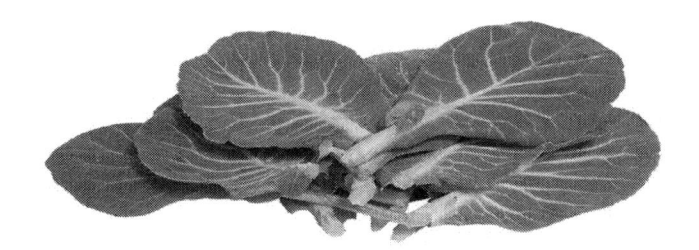

Take the washed collard greens and lay them flat. First put the spread of your choice in the middle of the leaf then put some of each of the rest of the ingredients and wrap like a burrito! Yum these are so good and good for you too!

CRUNCHY LETTUCE WRAPS

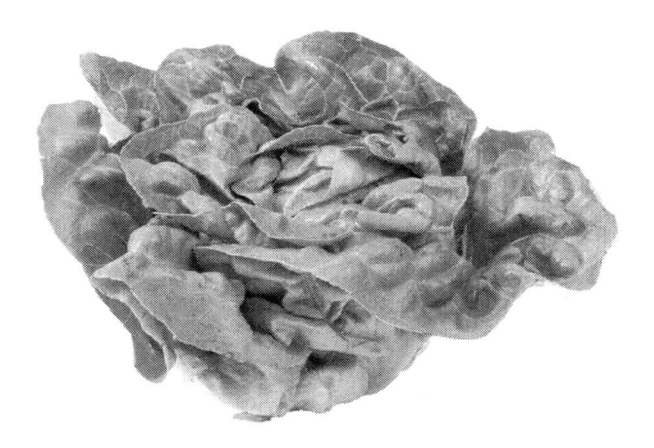

A small head of bib lettuce or romaine (cleaned and washed)
1 cup jicama (peeled and sliced into thin 1 inch pieces)
½ cup cilantro cleaned (not chopped; just kept in single strands)
1 cup thinly sliced red peppers
2 cup of bean sprouts
1/2 cup chopped raw peanuts (for top)
½ cup lime peanut sauce (this is a simple sauce of raw peanut butter mixed with lime juice to the consistency of a thin sauce)

Take the bib lettuce or romaine (I like bib because it is a little softer and easier to handle when you are eating it) and put some of each ingredient inside and wrap it up and serve with either the peanut sauce or put the peanut sauce inside the wrap. I like it with both!

SWEET NORI WRAPS

1 cup strawberries thinly sliced
1 cup papaya thinly sliced
1 cup mango thinly sliced
$\frac{1}{4}$ cup mint leaves whole
Cashew dipping sauce, which is 1 cup cashews soaked for 4 hours and then drained. Put the soaked cashews into a vita mixer along with 2 tablespoons of lime juice, and 1 tablespoon of agave nectar, and a small amount of water or $\frac{1}{2}$ an orange squeezed to make the right consistency for a sauce.

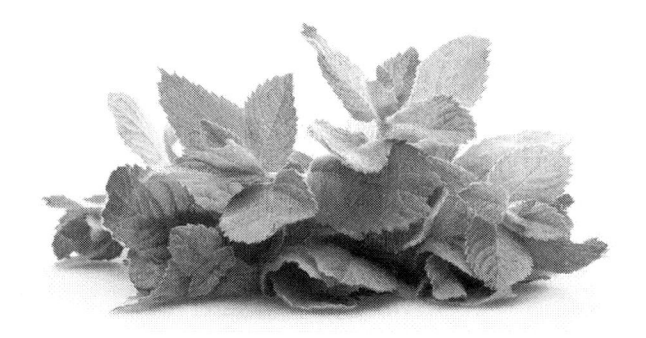

Keep the nori sheets dry on a cutting board and start to fill the nori at the end that is closest to you with the fruits and then start rolling the nori up. After that you will slice the nori into smaller sushi style pieces and dip the pieces into the dipping sauce.

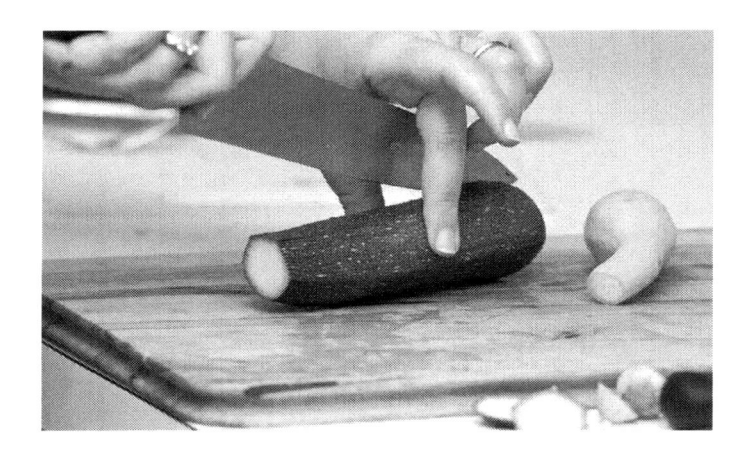

VEGGIE NORI WRAPS

1 cup thinly sliced zucchini
1 cup thinly sliced carrots
1 cup thinly sliced red pepper
2 avocados
1 cup thinly sliced cucumber
1 cup of basil leaves

Take the vegetables and clean and peel them then take the carrot, red pepper, and cucumber and make thin slices the length of the vegetable. Take the avocados and deseed them and mash them up into a spread.

Again keep the nori sheets dry and start and the end closest to you and put a thin layer of the avocado spread on the beginning of the nori sheet, then some of each of the other veggies and then roll it, slice it, and eat it! You can use Braggs for a dipping sauce if you like or whatever you like best.

SUN DRIED TOMATO & ARUGULA PIZZA

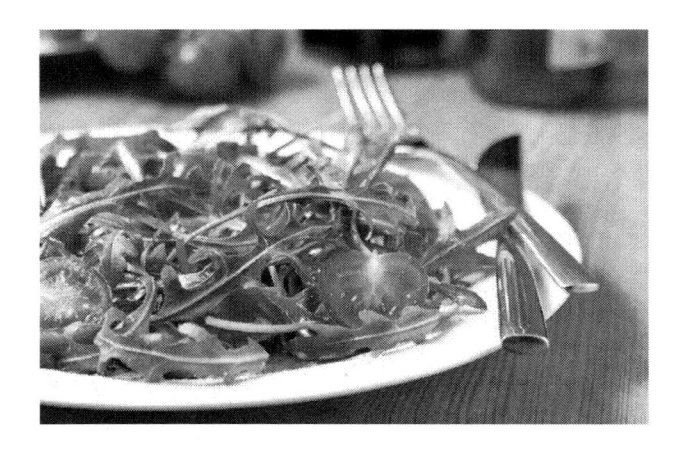

2 CUPS OF ARUGULA
1 CUP SUNDRIED TOMATO SPREAD (WHICH IS $\frac{3}{4}$ CUP OF SUNDRIED TOMATOES SOAKED AND DRAINED. USING A VITAMIXER GRIND UP THE

SUNDRIED TOMATOES ALONG WITH ¼ CUP OLIVE OIL, SALT AND PEPPER, ¼ CUP RAW PINE NUTS & HALF OF THE BASIL)
4-5 SEED, FLAX, ETC DEHYDRATED CRACKERS OF YOUR LIKING. YOU CAN PURCHASE THESE IN MOST HEALTH FOOD STORES OR IF YOU FEEL AMBITIOUS YOU CAN ALSO MAKE THEM YOURSELF!
¼ CUP BASIL

TAKE THE FLAX CRACKERS AND SPREAD THE SUNDRIED TOMATO SPREAD ON THE TOP. TAKE THE ARUGULA AND THE REST OF THE BASIL AND MIX IT WITH A LITTLE BALSAMIC AND OLIVE OIL (JUST ENOUGH TO BARELY COAT THE ARUGULA) AND THEN PUT THE ARUGULA ON TOP OF THE SUN DRIED TOMATO SPREAD AND YOUR DONE! THIS IS A GREAT TREAT. YOU CAN ALSO USE OTHER ITEMS LIKE TOMATOES SLICED, GREEN PEPPERS, RED PEPPERS, ETC.

MUSHROOM & TOMATO PESTO PIZZA

4-5 flax, Italian, etc dehydrated crackers
Pesto sauce (1 cup walnuts soaked for 4-5 hours and drained, 1 cup basil leaves, ¼-1/2 cup of olive oil, 1/8 cup lime juice 1 clove of garlic and salt and pepper to

taste. Using the vita mixer grind all of the ingredients together to a smooth consistency (you may need a little water or extra olive oil it will just depend).
1 cup sliced tomatoes
1 cup sliced crimini mushrooms

Take the Italian crackers and spread the raw pesto on the top and then add the sliced tomatoes and mushrooms and sprinkle with basil.

MEDITERRANEAN BURRITOS

2 cups sprouted garbanzo beans (see my website www.rawfoodfortoday.com) or soak the beans for 8 hours and allow to sprout for 2-3 days
1/2 cup olive oil
¼ cup raw tahini butter

6-8 bib lettuce leaves not broken
1 cup sliced cucumbers in 1 inch pieces
1 cup red peppers sliced into 1 inch pieces
1 cup diced tomatoes
1 bunch of chopped cilantro
Salt and pepper

In a food processor combine garbanzo beans, tahini butter, olive oil, and salt and pepper and blend until smooth. Next spread the garbanzo bean mixture on the inside of the bib lettuce and arrange the raw veggies and wrap it up and eat it! This is great because you can put all kinds of veggies in these and change it up a little more.

ALFREDO RAW PASTA

3-4 medium yellow zucchini use a spiral slicer and slice all of the zucchini into long spirals
2 cups of raw cashews soaked for 4-6 hours
¼ cup olive oil
1 clove of garlic
½ cup of lemon juice
Salt and pepper
¼ cup of basil
1/8 cup of Bragg's amino acids

This is one of my favorite meals! I love this! Once you have the zucchini sliced put it in a large bowl. Now take the soaked cashews and drain them and put the cashews and the rest of the ingredients into a vita mixer and blend until it is a smooth sauce. Next put the sauce on the zucchini and sprinkle with basil.

PESTO LINGUINI

3-4 zucchini or squash
2 cups raw walnuts nuts soaked for 4-6 hours
1 ½ cups of basil
½ cup oil
Salt and pepper
Clove of garlic

Start with taking the zucchini or squash and cutting it into a large square by cutting the skin off. Then cut that in half and take a peeler and make strips out of both halves so that they look like fettuccini. Then take the walnuts and drain them but save the water in case you need more liquid for the sauce and then add the rest of the ingredients and blend into a sauce. Then take the pesto and toss the zucchini with it and you are done. You can add sliced red peppers if you like to add more color and nutrition. It's all up to you.

SPAGHETTI SQUASH WITH SPICY GARLIC SAUCE

1 whole spaghetti squash
Sliced carrots
Sliced green zucchini
1 clove of garlic
½ cup of olive oil
½ teaspoon of red chili peppers
Salt and pepper

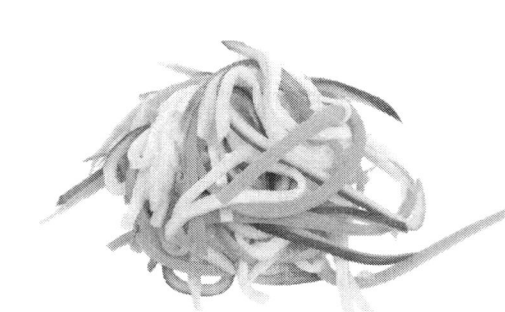

This recipe is so easy you will wonder why you don't eat this everyday! First you put the olive oil, chopped garlic, chili peppers, and salt and pepper into a small bowl to blend the flavors. Then you cut the squash in half and then start to scrap the squash out so that there are strings of the squash that look like spaghetti. I use a spoon with sharp points on the end so that it breaks up the squash better. Then you put the squash in a bowl and toss it with the olive oil mixture. If you want you can add slivered red peppers or chopped tomatoes to give the dish more color. If you don't like hot dishes you can also omit the chili peppers. It's really up to your taste buds.

ITALIAN CAPRESE TOWERS

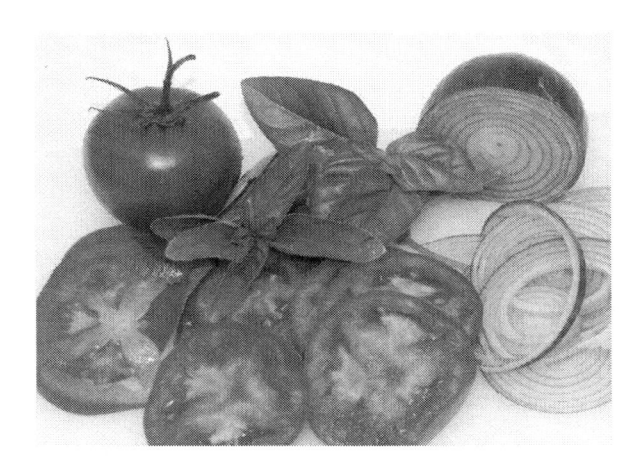

3-4 large heirloom tomatoes
Sliced onion (whichever kind you like best)
2 cups sliced marinated Portobello's (in a bowl soak the sliced mushrooms in ½ cup balsamic vinegar, ½ cup tamari, and ¼ cup olive oil for 4-6 hours)
Pesto from recipe number 9
Raw ricotta

First slice the tomatoes. On a large plate arrange the ingredients in layers starting with the tomatoes, then pesto, then portabellas, then raw ricotta (which is 2 cups raw pine nuts, salt and pepper, 3 tablespoons of lemon juice, 1 tablespoon of nutritional yeast, and a couple teaspoons of olive oil. Place all ingredients in a food processor until combined well) and finally the onion. Keep building little towers on the large plate so that everyone gets one or two.

LASAGNA

4-5 thinly sliced zucchini
3-4 cups marinated Portobello's (recipe 11)
Raw ricotta (in recipe 11)
6-8 medium tomatoes
1 cup chopped basil
1 clove of garlic
¼ cup olive oil
1 tablespoon oregano or Italian spices

First start by making the tomato sauce. Using a vita mixer put the tomatoes, basil, garlic, olive oil spices, and salt and pepper and blend until it looks like a nice thick sauce. Now take a glass baking dish and start to layer the thinly sliced zucchini, then ricotta sauce, tomato sauce, and then start another layer using the portabellas mushrooms, ricotta, and then sauce. Keep doing this until all of the ingredients are used up and top with some freshly chopped basil.

STUFFED TOMATOES

7-8 large tomatoes
1 cup chopped basil
1 clove garlic
1/8 cup of olive oil
Salt and pepper
1 large jicama peeled
1 cup raw pine nuts soaked for 2 hours

First take all of the tomatoes and cut into halves. Then scoop out the inside of the tomatoes and then place them in a large glass baking sheet. Next take the rest of the ingredients and blend in a food processor (leaving out ½ cup of the basil for garnish) until smooth and then fill the tomatoes with the filling and top with basil and serve!

RAVIOLI

1 eggplant sliced into very thin rounds with a mandoline
Raw ricotta (on page 151)
Pesto sauce (on page 149)

Place the thinly sliced eggplant in a bowl of water with 1 tablespoon of salt and let soak for 2 hours, then drain and pat dry. Now add the raw ricotta and fold in half and drizzle with olive oil and pesto sauce. You can use other raw sauces if you would like such as marinara, sun dried tomato, etc.

QUINOA SUMMER SALAD

1 cup sprouted quinoa (soak for 2 hours and let sprout for 1 day)
¼ cup chopped mint
1 cup cucumber diced into small pieces
1 cup red and green peppers chopped into small pieces
½ cup chopped parsley
1 clove of garlic chopped fine
½ cup olive oil
½ cup lemon juice
Salt and pepper

Mix all ingredients in a bowl and serve.

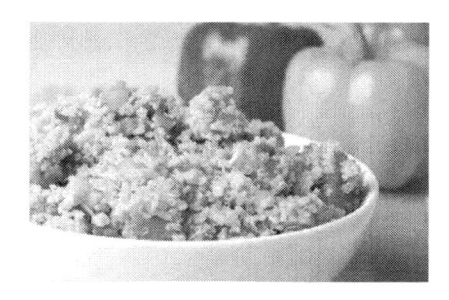

THAI WILD RICE SALAD

2 cups wild rice soaked for 9 hours and sprouted for 3-5 days
1 cup finely chopped celery
1 cup diced carrots
½ cup diced red pepper
1 teaspoon of ginger
1 clove of garlic chopped fine
1 cup chopped raw peanuts
1/2 cup chopped basil
1 tablespoon of raw almond butter
½ cup chopped cilantro
½-3/4 cup lime juice
¼ cup olive oil
Salt and pepper
Dash of chili peppers
Mix all ingredients together and serve.

SWEET SUMMER WILD RICE SALAD

1. Cups wild rice soaked for 9 hours and sprouted for 3-5 days
1 large red apple cut into small pieces
1 celery stalk cut into small pieces

1 cup of dried currants
1 cup chopped raw cashews
¼ cup chopped parsley
1 tablespoon of olive oil
1 teaspoon of agave nectar
Salt and pepper
Mix all ingredients in a bowl and serve.

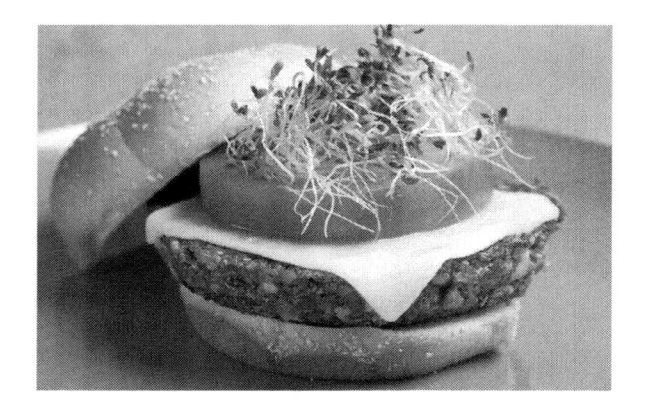

RAW BURGER

2   Cups of raw walnuts
2   Cups carrots
     ¼ cup celery
1   Clove of garlic
     1 shallot
     1 teaspoon of agave nectar
     1 pitted date
     1 tablespoon of olive oil

1 tablespoon of Italian seasoning
Salt and pepper

Mix all ingredients in a food processor until blended. The mixture should be easily shaped into round patties. Then dress with sliced tomatoes, onions, cucumbers, etc.

LENTIL SALAD

2 cups lentils soaked for 7 hours and sprouted for 3 days
1/2 cup lemon juice
1 cup chopped parsley
1 cup small diced tomatoes
$\frac{1}{4}$ cup olive oil
Salt and pepper
1 teaspoon of cumin

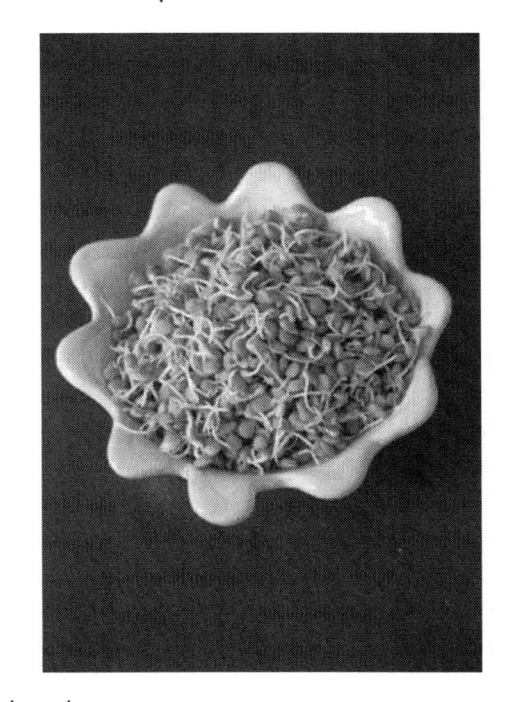

Mix all ingredients in a bowl and serve.

ITALIAN BARLEY SALAD

2 cups barley soaked for 6 hours and sprouted for 2 days
1 cup sundried tomatoes soaked for 4 hours
1 clove of garlic chopped fine
1 cup pitted and chopped black olives
½ cup chopped basil
¼-1/2 cup olive oil
Salt and pepper

DRAIN THE SUN DRIED TOMATOES AND CHOPPED INTO SMALL PIECES. TAKE THE REST OF THE INGREDIENTS AND MIX IN A BOWL AND SERVE.

20 Raw Desserts

Apple Tartlet

Lemon Cookies

Coconut Haystacks

Cherry Crisp

Raw Key Lime Pudding

Almond Butter Bars

Apricot Cookies

Raw Pumpkin Pie

Raw Mango Pudding

Raw Banana Cream Pie

Raw Chocolate Chip Cookies

Raw Pecan Pie

Raw Chocolate Cream Pie

Raw Apple Pie

Raw Cheesecake

Raw Banana Chocolate Ice Cream

Raw Strawberry Ice Cream

Raw Rice Pudding

Chocolate Macadamia Pudding

Oatmeal Cookies

APPLE TARTLETS WITH CACAO BANANA SAUCE

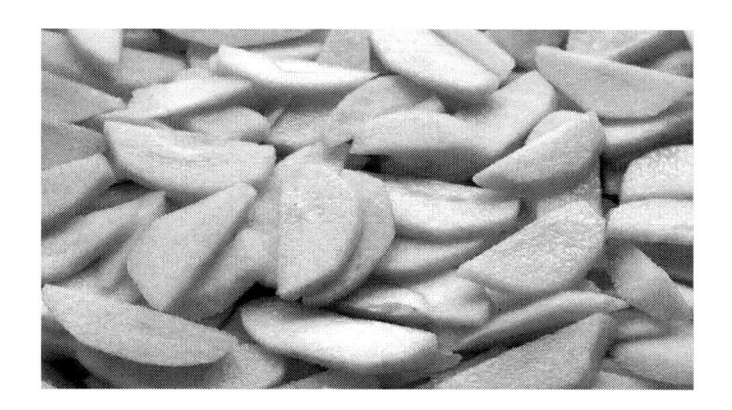

Serves 4

Crust:

3 cups young coconut, shredded & dehydrated
3 medjool dates (pitted)

Blend coconut in blender or food processor until fine and then add the dates and blend. Press into 4, 3 inch tartlet pans, lined with parchment paper. Freeze for 2 hours. Take out, discard liner, and let stand for 15 minutes before adding filling.

Filling:

4 cups apples, cored & peeled
½ Cup of Chopped Raw Almonds
1 tsp cinnamon
1/8 tsp nutmeg

1/4 tsp fresh ginger
2 tbsp lemon juice

Put apples in a food processor until chunky. Stir in lemon juice and spices. Pour into crust and top with chopped almond sauce.

Cacao Banana Sauce:

1 Half of Banana
2 tsp of raw Cacao powder
1 Young coconut
2 fresh medjool date

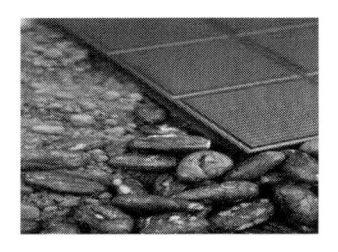

Carefully open up young coconuts and empty liquid into a Vita mixer blender. Scoop out white "meat" out of the coconut and put into blender as well. Add half of the banana, pitted dates, and cocoa powder into blender, blend until smooth.

Place tartlet on plate, spoon sauce on tartlet, and sprinkle chopped almonds on top.

LEMON COOKIES

2 cups raw cashews (not soaked)
2 cups shredded coconut
½ cup lemon juice
¼ Cup of almond milk
1/4 cup lemon zest
1/4 cup maple syrup

Blend all ingredients in a food processor until smooth and then form into cookie shapes and dehydrate for 12hours at 90 degrees.

COCONUT HAYSTACKS

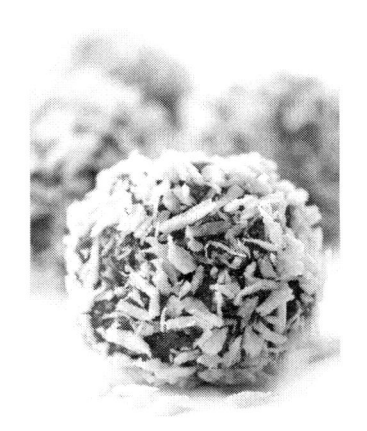

1 Cup coconut oil
½ Cup raw honey
¼ Cup maple syrup
½ Cup cocoa powder
1 teaspoon vanilla extract
4 Cups shredded coconut

Blend all ingredients except the shredded coconut in a food processor until smooth. Next add the coconut to the mixture and form into round balls and place on parchment paper and freeze. They will become soft if left out of the freezer for very long so bring them out around 15 minutes before serving.

CHERRY CRISP

Yield: 1 (8-inch) crisp

Crumble Topping:
2 cups raw walnuts or pecans chopped
½ cup raw oats
1/2 cup unsweetened shredded dried coconut
1/4 teaspoon ground cinnamon
1/4 teaspoon ground nutmeg
1/4 teaspoon salt
1/2 cup dried cherries chopped
8 pitted medjool dates ground up small
1/4 cup maple syrup

Filling:
30 oz of frozen cherries frozen thawed and drained
3/4 cup pitted medjool dates, soaked
1 tablespoon fresh lemon juice

Blend all of the filling and put into a glass baking container. Then take the crumble topping and mix by hand until smooth and then put the crumble on top of the cherries.

RAW KEY LIME PUDDING

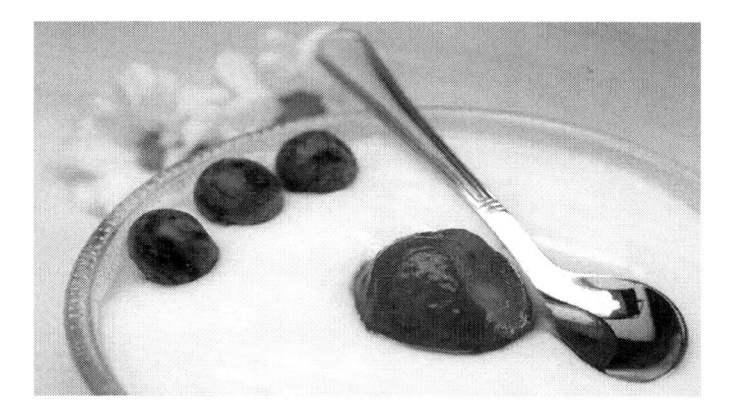

1 cup young coconut meat
2 tablespoons coconut butter
½ cup macadamia nuts
¼ cup coconut water
4 tablespoons key lime juice
1 key lime for zesting
¼ teaspoon Celtic sea salt
1 Tablespoon of maple syrup

Mix the macadamia nuts, water, coconut water and lime juice in a high-powered blender, vita mixer, or food processor and blend until smooth. Then add all other ingredients and blend until smooth. Refrigerate for at least 1 hour before serving so that pudding may thicken. Then top with key lime zest.

ALMOND BUTTER BARS

3/4 cup raw almond butter
1/4 cup Macadamia nut butter
1/2 cup raw honey
1 cup raw sesame seeds
1/4 cup of raw cacao powder
1/2 cup of shredded coconut

Mix all ingredients in a food processor on slow and then remove and put into a glass pan and then top with chopped raw almonds!

APRICOT COOKIE

2 Cups oats soaked
2 Cups dried apricots
1 Cup of dates pitted
½ Cup dried figs soaked
1 Cup finely ground flaxseeds
1 Cup pecans chopped
½ Cup maple syrup
(Save the water from soaking the figs)

In a vita mixer add the oats, dates, dried figs; soak water, finely ground flaxseeds, and maple syrup. Take the mixture and add the chopped apricots and chopped pecans and form into cookies and dehydrate for 100 degrees for 4 hours on each side.

RAW PUMPKIN PIE

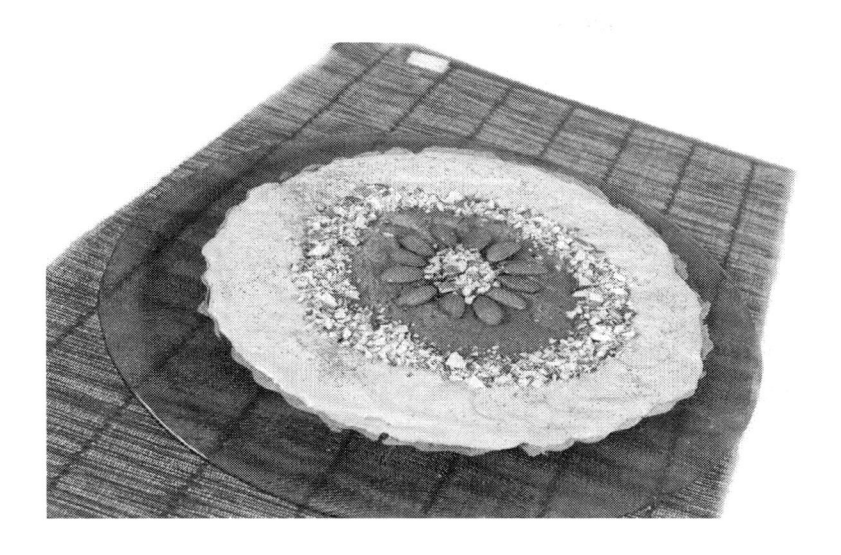

Crust:
1 Cup raw pecans ground up fine
1 Tbsp. lemon zest
6 dates pitted
Mix all ingredients in a food processor until smooth and then spread out evenly in dish.

Filling

2 Cups Raw Pumpkin cut up
1 Avocado pitted

1 Tbsp Lemon Juice
2 Teaspoons of pumpkin spices
2 Tablespoons of maple syrup
2 Tablespoon of finely ground flaxseeds
1/2 Teaspoon Fresh Ginger

Put all ingredients in food processor and process until smooth. Put into dish onto crust and spread evenly. Set in
Fridge to allow to set some more. Serve with following whip.

Whip:

1 Cup of Macadamia Nuts
7 Pitted Dates
1 Tbsp. Lemon Juice
2-3 Tablespoons of orange juice

Put all ingredients in Blender and let process until smooth. Keep adding the orange juice to keep the mixture thin enough to whip in the blender.

You want the whip to be smooth and thick but loose enough to just about pour.

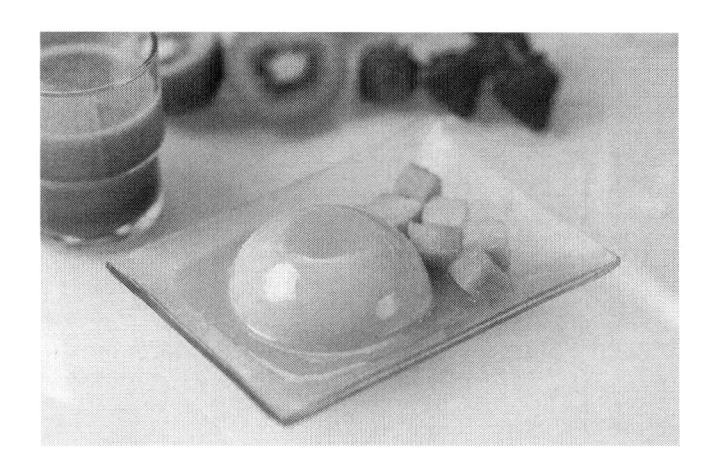

RAW MANGO PUDDING

2 Mangos
1 Cup of macadamia nuts soaked for 4 hours
1 Cup young coconut meat
1/8 Cup of lime juice
Shredded Coconut & Chopped macadamia nuts for the topping.

Use a vegetable peeler to peel mangos. Then cut the mango into pieces throwing away the pit. Drain the macadamia nuts and put all the ingredients in a blender and blend until smooth. Then add shredded coconut and chopped macadamia to taste.

RAW BANANA COCONUT CREAM PIE

For the Crust:

1 Cup Macadamia Nuts
½ Cup Shredded Dry Coconut
1 tsp Coconut Oil
2 Tablespoons of Raw Honey
Pinch of Salt

For the Filling:

2 Cups Young Coconut Meat About 2 young coconuts
½ Cup Raw Coconut Oil
3 Tablespoons of Raw Honey
2 Tablespoon Lime Juice
¼ teaspoon Salt
½ teaspoon Vanilla Extract
3 bananas (2 of them sliced)

Preparing The Crust
Blend first 5 ingredients in a food processor then add more honey if needed to make crust sticky. Line pie pan with saran wrap and press crust on top. Place in freezer while making the filling.

Preparing the Filling
Blend the rest of the ingredients, (**except bananas that are sliced**) in a vita mixer until smooth.
Make sure there is enough liquid to have the ingredients moving, you may need to add coconut water. Take crust out from freezer and place sliced bananas on top of crust. Pour filling on top of bananas. Place in freezer for 3-4 hours to set.

Top with shredded coconut! Yum

RAW "CHOCOLATE CHIP" COOKIES

1 cup raw walnuts
1 Cup Pecans
1 Cup Macadamia Nuts
15 dates
1 Teaspoon of cinnamon
½ tsp salt
2 Tablespoon raw coconut oil
4 tablespoons cacao nibs

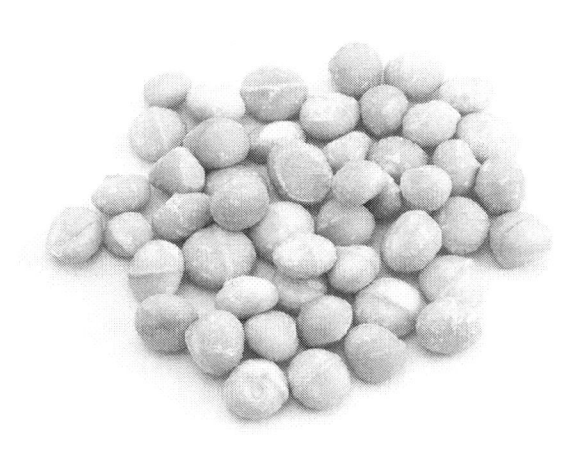

Place dates in food processor and mix until smooth. Add nuts, cinnamon, salt and coconut oil and mix it all up, again until smooth. Once smooth, add cacao nibs and blend just until nibs are well distributed. After ingredients are mixed, remove from food processor and use a spoon to make flat cookie shapes. Refrigerate before eating.

RAW PECAN PIE

For the crust:

1 Cup Macadamia Nuts
½ Cup Shredded Dry Coconut
1 tsp Coconut Oil
2 Tablespoons of Raw Honey
Pinch of Salt

For the filling:

- 2 Cups pecans processed in a food processor until smooth
- 30 pitted dates
- 2 Cups shredded, dried coconut
- 1/2 teaspoon salt
- 1 teaspoon cinnamon
- 1/2 cup pecans, chopped

Preparing the Crust

Blend first 5 ingredients in a food processor then add more honey if needed to make crust sticky. Line pie pan with saran

wrap and press crust on top.
Place in freezer while making the
filling.

For the Filling:

In food processor, process dates until smooth (or as close to smooth as you can get). Add the smooth pecans, coconut, salt, and cinnamon. Process until everything is well mixed. Remove from food processor and then place ingredients in the prepared crust. Top with the extra chopped pecans and then refrigerate for 1-2 hours.

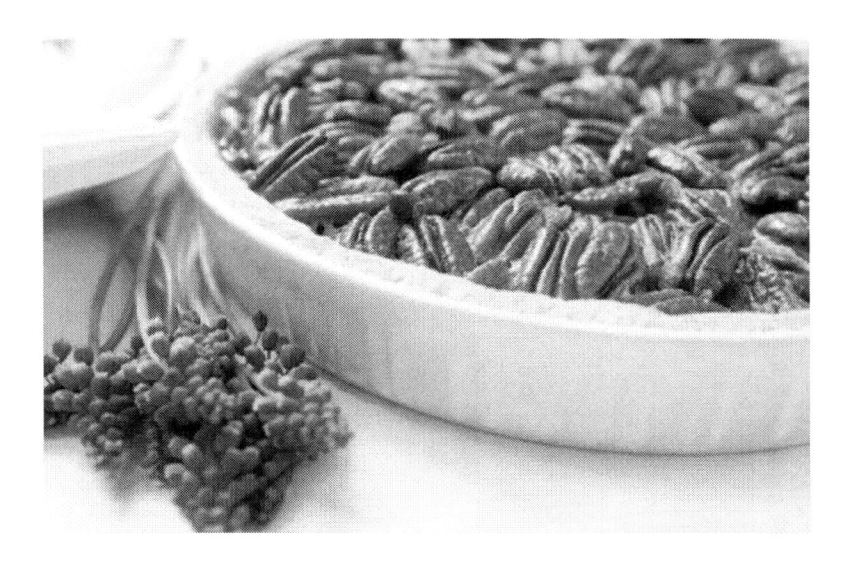

RAW CHOCOLATE CREAM PIE

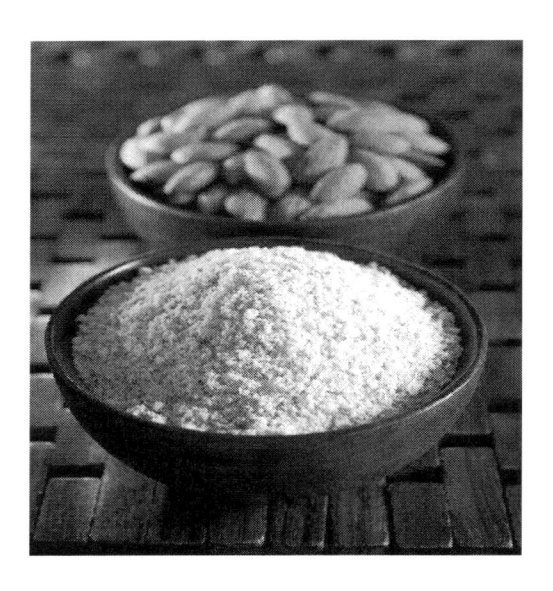

Crust
1/2 Cup Almonds
1/2 Cup Pecans
1/2 Cup of Brazil Nuts
 8 Pitted Dates
1/4 Cup Agave Syrup
1/4 Cup Cacao Powder
Pinch Sea Salt

Put nuts into food processor and process until ground. Place the rest of the ingredients in processor with nuts and process until combined. Spread onto a pie pan using your hands.

Cream Filling

Meat of 2 Young Thai Coconuts
2 Avocado
6 Pitted Dates
1/2 Cup Cacao Powder
2 Tablespoons of Maple syrup

Place all ingredients in food processor and process until well combined. If filling is not sweet or chocolaty enough for you add a more syrup or more cacao powder respectively. Spread into inside of pie crust. Top with some sliced strawberries or raspberries for added flavor.
Chill in refrigerator for 1-2 hours and serve.

RAW APPLE PIE

Crust:

1 ½ Cups of raw almonds soaked for 4-6 hours
1/8 Cup of Olive Oil
1 Tablespoon of coconut oil
Pinch of salt

Filling:

4-5 Red apples cored
5 Pitted dates
1 teaspoon of coconut oil
2 Tablespoons of maple syrup
1 teaspoon of cinnamon
Pinch of salt

Blend the almonds in a food processor and then add the rest of the crust ingredients. Put the crust into a glass pie pan. Next take the filling ingredients and blend together and pour into the crust pan. Chill in the refrigerator for 1-2 hours.

RAW CHEESECAKE

The Crust
2 Cups Raw macadamia nuts
8 Pitted dates
¼ cup dried coconut

Filling:

3 Cups cashews soaked for at least 3 hours
¾ Cup lemon juice
¾ cups maple syrup
¾ Cup coconut oil
Meat from one raw young coconut
½ cup cocoa nibs

Make the crust by processing the ingredients in a food processor. Press the ingredients into a spring form pan. Next blend the cashews, lemon, maple syrup, coconut oil, young coconut meat, vanilla, and sea salt. Blend until smooth. Pour the mixture onto the crust and top with cocoa nibs and then freeze until firm.

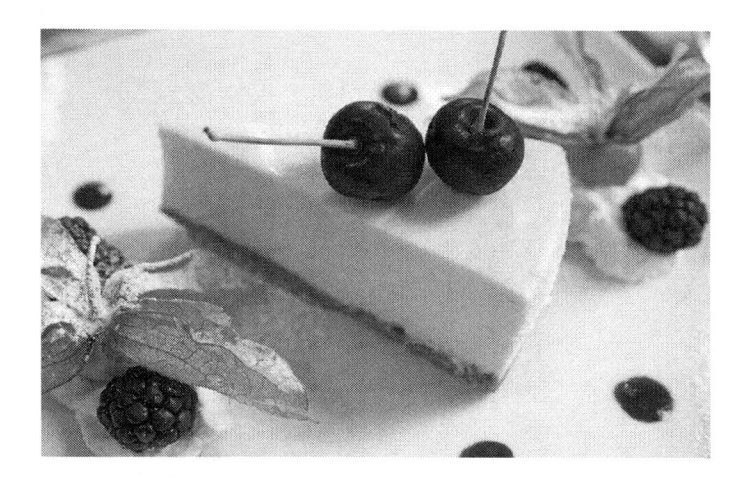

RAW BANANA & CHOCOLATE ICE CREAM

3 bananas sliced and then frozen
¼ c raw cacao or cocoa powder
2 T raw honey
1 teaspoon vanilla
1 pinch of salt
¼ cup cocoa nibs

Remove bananas from freezer and place them in a food processor; add cacao, honey, salt and vanilla and mix until thick and creamy. Add cocoa nibs and blend quickly, just until they are mixed through, but not ground too small. Pour mixture into a loaf pan and cover with saran wrap. Place in freezer. When serving, remove from freezer 5 minutes before. Scoop and serve, just as you would regular ice cream.

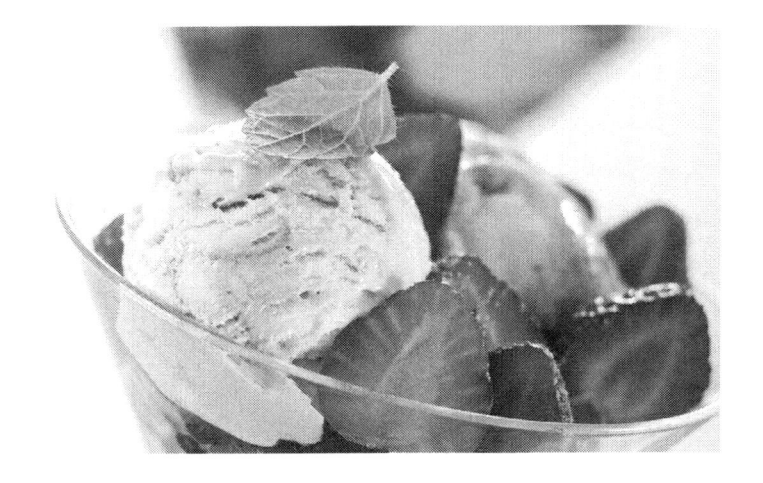

RAWBERRY ICE CREAM

1 Frozen banana
1 Cup fresh strawberries
$\frac{1}{4}$ Cup raw honey
The meat from one raw coconut
2 Cups raw cashews
Pinch of salt

Blend all ingredients in a food processor until smooth and then place in a container and freeze.

RAW RICE PUDDING

1 ½ Cup of brown rice soaked for 3 days
4 Young coconuts
2 teaspoons of cinnamon
1 teaspoon of nutmeg
1 teaspoon of vanilla
2 Tablespoons of maple syrup

In a vita mixer blend the coconut meat and only 2 cups of the coconut water, cinnamon, vanilla, and maple syrup. Blend until smooth. In a large bowl mix in the rice and the blended ingredients and let set in the refrigerator for 1 hour.

CHOCOLATE MACADAMIA PUDDING

2 Cups Raw macadamia nuts
2 Cups pitted dates
½ cup cocoa powder
1 Cup of coconut water

Blend all ingredients together until smooth and serve.

RAW OATMEAL COOKIES

2 Cups Oats Soaked overnight
1/2 Cup of Almond milk

10 pitted dates
1 Cup of raw almonds
½ Cup Raisons
½ Cup Maple Syrup

Mix all ingredients in a food processor (except the raisons) and blend. Next add the raisons. Now take small amounts of the dough and flatten on a dehydrator sheets so they resemble cookies and dehydrate for 12 hours at 110 degrees. Yum!

Thanks for taking the time to try these healthy recipes. You will be glad you did. Also I would like to take a minute to tell you how important it is to purchase organic produce.

Why eat organic?

Eating organic is a choice that most of us ponder every day. I know I always chose organic when I can or when I have enough money. But what does organic mean? The first organic produce law was in 1990 from congress and it stated that food grown without pesticides, fungicides, or not genetically modified would be considered organic. Pesticides are toxic and bad for the environment, farmers, and for you and your family. Genetically modified food (food that is made to be larger, better coloring, and pest resistant) has been questioned by many people. No one really knows the long-term effects of this on your body.

Some of the highest levels of pesticide residue on produce that is considered not organic are apricots, nectarines, green beans, potatoes, bananas, cucumbers, celery, corn, peppers, cherries, apples, spinach, tomatoes, soy beans, rice, strawberries, dates, carrots, grapes, peaches, pears, lemons, milk, and sweet potatoes. So I guess if you don't eat any of these your o.k. well that sounds like a lot of fruits and vegetables to me. There have been numerous studies showing how foods grown without pesticides and fungicides have more nutritional value and a much higher mineral content. Even if the nutritional level was a little better don't you think that you would want that for you and your family? It is also very important to drink organic milk or milk products that have been made without growth hormone and antibiotics. I think I will take my antibiotics from the doctor thank you!

Some ways to get more organic produce in your daily diet is to shop at local farmers markets, ask your local supermarket to carry more organic choices, at the seasonal farmers markets buy extra so you can dehydrate or freeze your extras for the winter months, start a garden, order online and have it delivered, become a member of a food co-op, start a food co-op, or participate in a organic food buying club. These are some simple ways to introduce organic food into you and your family's diet. You and your family are worth it. The more demand in the market place for organic produce the soy beans, rice, strawberries, dates, carrots, grapes, peaches, pears, lemons, milk, and sweet potatoes. So I guess if you don't eat any of these your o.k. well that sounds like a lot of fruits and vegetables to me. There have been numerous studies showing how foods grown without pesticides and fungicides have more nutritional value and a much higher mineral content. Even if the nutritional level was a little better don't you think that you would want that for you and your family? It is also very important to drink organic milk or milk products that have been made without growth hormone and antibiotics. I think I will take my antibiotics from the doctor thank you!

Some ways to get more organic produce in your daily diet is to shop at local farmers markets, ask your local supermarket to carry more organic choices, at the seasonal farmers markets buy extra so you can dehydrate or freeze your extras for the winter months, start a garden, order online and have it delivered, become a member of a food co-op, start a food co-op, or participate in a organic food buying club. These are some simple ways to introduce organic food into you and your family's diet. You and your family are worth it. The more demand in the market place for organic produce the cheaper it will eventually be. Do your part in helping the environment and support your local farmers. It only takes a few people in every town to make a difference. Let it be you!

About the Author:

B.S. Science in Physical Anthropology minor in business, and Culinary Arts Degree.

Advocate for organic, vegetarian, vegan, raw food diets, writing, yoga, swimming, biking, and running 5 K's! I have been a vegetarian/vegan/raw foodist for over 20 years. I have also worked in real estate for over ten years and have several websites to help people who are interested in raw food http://www.Recipes4RawFood.com and http://www.RawFoodForToday.com .

I have also started the Raw Foods Association with my husband so that others can become members of a larger healthy group and its website is www.RawFoodsAssociation.com!

For more information on how to order books, original articles, become a member of the Raw Foods Association, and updates on future projects go to www.rawfoodfortoday.com. www.sunnycabanapublishing.com, or www.recipes4rawfood.com!

RECIPES 4 RAW FOOD

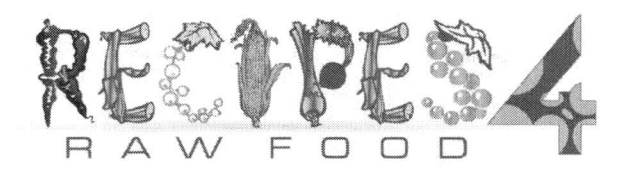

1314 E Las Olas Blvd

Fort Lauderdale, FL 33301

Recipes4RawFood@yahoo.com

I hope you enjoy my raw recipes!

Check out more of my recipes at www.recipes4rawfood.com and www.rawfoodfortoday.com

If you have any suggestions, comments, or corrections please feel free to email me at recipes4rawfood@yahoo.com.

Other Sources for Raw Food Info:

Other helpful websites for raw food information are www.rawfoodsassociation.com , which has a directory of raw businesses and raw restaurants in your area.

www.veganmainstream.com Very helpful website for vegan businesses. They also have a wonderful blog to follow in order to gain more information on the raw food industry. I highly recommend this site to any new vegan or raw business.

www.yogastudiosusa.com is another great site if you are traveling and would like to find a yoga studio.

One of my favorite ways to get connected to the raw food or yoga community is to join a raw or yoga group on www.meetup.com.

Raw Education or Raw Retreats

Arizona

Tree of Life Rejuvenation Center
PO Box 1080
Patagonia, AZ 85624
www.treeoflife.nu
healing@treeoflife.nu

California

Healing for Bliss
PO Box 417
Ojai, CA 93024
www.healingforbliss.com
info@helaingforbliss.com

Living Light Culinary Arts Institute
704 N Harrison
Fort Bragg, CA 95437
www.rawfoodchef.com
info@rawfoodchef.com

Optimum Health Institute of San Diego
6970 Central Ave
Lemon Grove, CA 91945

www.optimumhealth.org

Colorado & California

Bauman College
www.baumancollege.org
Four Locations
Pennegrove, CA
Berkley, CA
Santa Cruz, CA
Boulder, CO

Florida

Hippocrates Health Institute
1443 Palmdale Court
West Palm Beach, FL
561-471-8876

Circle of Life Retreat
PO Box 604
Delray Beach, FL 33447
561-638-8873
jayneschneider@earthlink.net

Georgia

The Living Foods Institute
1530 Dekalb Ave. NE Ste E
Atlanta, GA 30307
www.livingfoodsinstiture.com
info@livingfoodsinstiture.com

Illinois

Cousins Incredible Vitality
3038 W Irving Park Rd
Chicago, IL 60618
info@cousinsiv.com
773-478-6868

Michigan
Creative Health Institute
918 Union City Rd
Union City, MI 49094
517-278-6260

New Mexico

Ann Wigmore Foundation
PO Box 399

San Sidel, NM 87049
www.annwigmore.org
505-552-0595

New York

The First Supper
108 Forest Ave
Glen Cove Long Island, NY
www.thefirstsupper.com
516-759-2606

Oklahoma

105 Degrees Academy
5820 N Classen Blvd Ste 1
Oklahoma City, OK 73118
contact@105degrees.com
www.105degrees.com
405-842-1050

Oregon

Hummingbird Homestead
22732 NW Gilliham Rd
Sauvie Island, OR 97231

jayne@earthworld.com

Puerto Rico

Ann Wigmore Institute
Ruta 115. KM 20
Barrio Guayabo
Aguada, PR 00743
info@annwigmore.org
787-868-6307

Texas

Optimum Health Institute of Austin
264 Cedar Lane
Cedar Creek, TX 78612
512-303-4817

Raw Dolphins Residential Retreats
Bimini Bay Resort and Spa
Bimini/Atlantis
www.rawdolphins.com
rawdolphins@live.com
Yoga and raw food retreat!

Canada
New Life Retreat
RR4, 453 Dobbie Rd
Lanark, Ontario K0G 1K0
613-259-3337

Simply Raw
www.simplyraw.ca
613-234-0806
Raw Foundation Culinary Arts Institute
6623 Nelson Ave
West Vancouver, BC
info@rawfoundation.ca
778-839-8424

Index

A

Acia Page 10, 63
Agave Nectar Page 68, 83, 109, 112, 123-128, 130, 131, 156
Aloe Vera Page 59, 66, 73
Almonds Page 29, 47, 87, 161, 162, 166, 174, 176, 179
Apples Page 24, 107, 124, 161, 175, 181
Apricot Page 166, 181
Arugula Page 119, 123, 124, 128, 139, 145, 146
Asparagus Page 97, 133
Avocados Page 10, 79, 80, 90, 91, 92, 101, 102, 124, 133, 134, 144, 145

B

Bananas Page 24, 62, 115, 170, 177, 181
Barley Page 34, 140, 158
Basil Page 45, 83, 84, 86, 97, 104, 110, 133, 144, 146-149, 152, 153, 155, 158
Beets Page 91, 130, 135
Blueberries Page 59, 62, 71, 76
Broccoli Page 29, 33, 120, 134
Burgers Page 139, 156
Burritos Page 90, 139, 147
Butternut Squash Page 111

C

Carrots Page 79, 96, 105, 109, 130, 141, 144, 150, 181
Cashews Page 47, 79, 83, 84, 88, 96, 109, 123, 143, 148, 156, 162, 176, 178
Celery Page 23, 24, 60, 61, 63, 65, 66, 72, 99, 101, 107, 108, 109, 115, 117, 155, 156, 181
Cheesecake Page 159, 176
Cherry Page 31, 57, 69, 120, 136, 159, 164

Chilies Page 44, 111
Chocolate Page 57, 68, 159, 171, 174, 171, 179
Cilantro Page 22, 77, 82,85, 86, 87, 89-91, 93, 95, 101-103, 105, 106, 110, 111, 115-117, 121, 142, 147, 155
Coconut Page 5, 10, 13, 39, 63, 64, 68, 69, 74, 78, 86, 87, 96, 99, 102, 105, 116, 159, 161-166, 169-173, 175, 176, 178
Collard Greens Page 82, 141
Cookies Page 159, 162, 166, 171, 179, 180
Cucumbers Page 31, 79, 101, 112, 118, 128, 129, 130, 131, 141, 147, 157, 181
Curry Page 78, 86, 96, 111, 115

D
Dates Page 43, 68, 73, 74, 114, 131, 132, 161, 162, 164, 166-168, 171-176, 179, 181
Dehydrator Page 24
Desserts Page 24, 159
Dill Page 78, 96, 105, 120, 128, 135

E
Eggplant Page 97, 153, 154
Endive Page 119, 121

F

Fennel Page 99, 104, 119, 124
Figs Page 76, 166
Flaxseeds Page 166, 168
Food Processor Page 19

G

Garlic Page 45, 83, 84, 87, 90, 91, 96, 102, 104, 109, 115, 116, 120, 130, 133-135, 139, 146, 148, 149, 150, 152-158
Gazpacho Page 23, 99, 101
Ginger Page 45, 57, 71, 72, 75, 105, 106, 115, 117, 155, 162, 168
Grapefruit Page 17, 78, 91-93, 123, 124
Green Tea Page 43, 57, 70

H

Hazelnuts Page 125
Habanera Page 44
Hemp Page 30, 37, 82, 95, 112, 121, 132

I

Ice Cream Page 159, 177, 178

J

Jalapenos Page 44
Jicama Page 77, 88, 93, 142, 153
Juicer Page 5, 13, 21

K

Kale Page 24, 29, 57, 62, 100, 117, 119, 122, 123
Kiwi Page 57, 66, 127
Knives Page 15

L

Lasagna Page 139, 152
Lentils Page 28, 33, 157
Lettuce Page 17, 31, 64, 69, 72, 117, 121, 131, 132, 139, 142, 147, 148
Lemon Page 9, 35, 84, 86, 87, 89, 99, 105-111, 117, 119, 121, 123, 128, 130-133, 135, 136, 148, 151, 157, 161, 164, 167, 168, 176, 181
Limes Page 85, 101, 102, 111

M

Macadamia Nuts Page 47, 48, 86, 96, 99, 108, 116, 131, 165-172, 176, 179
Mandoline Page 20, 153
Mangoes Page 57, 63, 77, 85, 99, 114, 143, 159, 169
Mint Page 113, 114, 119, 124, 131, 133, 143, 154
Mushrooms Page 77, 83, 85, 87, 139, 146, 151

N

Nectarine Page 58, 73, 181
Nori page 78, 94, 139, 144, 145
Nuts Page 25, 28, 36, 46-53, 84, 86, 89, 96, 108, 115, 125-127, 131, 134, 135, 142, 146, 149, 151, 153, 154, 162, 165, 168, 170, 172, 174, 176

O

Oats Page 35, 164, 166, 179
Oils Page 31, 36-39, 64, 79-81, 83, 85, 92, 93, 96, 97, 102, 106-112, 116, 121, 123-136, 146-154, 163, 170, 171, 175, 176.

Orange Page 22, 63-66, 69, 71, 72, 76, 79, 81, 93, 114, 115, 123, 124, 127, 128, 130, 131, 143, 168

P

Papaya Page 69, 143
Parsnip Page 136
Pasta Page 18, 148
Peas Page 29, 103, 131, 132
Peach Page 64, 181
Peanut Page 35, 111, 115, 133, 134, 142, 143, 155
Pear Page 72, 128
Pecans Page 47, 128, 133, 164, 167, 171, 173
Pesto Page 82, 141, 16, 147, 149, 151, 153, 154
Pies Page 41
Pine Nuts Page 84, 131, 146, 151, 153
Pizza Page 83, 139, 145
Plantains Page 81
Pomegranate Page 127
Pudding Page 165, 169, 178, 179
Pumpkin Page 35, 82, 136, 167, 168

Q

Quinoa Page 29, 34, 139, 154

R

Raisons Page 179, 180
Raspberries Page 125, 175
Ravioli Page 139, 153
Red Cabbage Page 135

Red Pepper Page 81, 85, 87, 89, 93, 95, 97, 102, 106, 121, 122, 134, 141, 146, 149, 155
Rice Page 139, 155, 178, 181
Romaine Page 64, 69-74, 79, 82, 99, 117, 136, 142

S

Smoothies Page 57
Soups Page 99
Spinach Page 31, 59, 60, 63, 65, 66, 73, 75, 76, 99, 112, 119, 126, 127, 181
Sprouts Page 27-35, 94, 14
Squash Page 99, 111, 135, 139, 149, 150
Strawberry Page 57, 60, 126
Sun Dried Tomato Page 79, 99, 110, 145, 158
Sweet and Salty Page 42
Sweet Potato Page 133, 134, 181

T

Thai Page 44, 86, 87, 105, 139, 155
Tomatoes Page 17, 22-24, 31, 35, 77, 79, 80, 83, 84, 88, 90, 91, 101, 102, 106, 109-111, 129, 130, 141, 145-147, 150-154, 157

U

V

Vegan Page 39, 47, 49, 184, 186
Vita Mixer Page 19, 59, 61, 62-76, 79, 82, 84, 88, 89, 90, 91, 96, 104, 108, 111-117, 130, 134-136, 143, 147, 148, 152, 162, 165, 166, 170, 179

W

Wakame Page 125, 126
Walnut Page 36, 47, 48, 89, 126-128, 135, 146, 149, 156, 164, 171
Wraps Page 82, 85, 94, 96, 141-144
Watermelon Page 106, 113, 119, 131

Y

Yoga Page 3, 10, 50-56

Z

Zucchini Page 18, 85, 86, 92, 93, 97, 115, 135, 144, 148-150, 152

Made in the USA
Lexington, KY
07 June 2019